THE ANCIENT RAW FOOD DIET
By
ROGER BEZANIS

Acknowledgements

*Without the aid and support of the following people, "The Ancient Raw Food Diet"
would not have come into existence. Stacy Brown, Suzi Ell, Darryl Sanford,
David and Carol Cintron, Micky "The Amazing", Ken Wright, "Mighty Morgan",
Jane Bosan, Dr. Ted Morter, Super Susanne, David Wolfe, and My Great Friend Ron.*

Neff / Harry Publishing © 2013
Cover Design & Graphics, Roger Bezanis and Susanne Abraham, SusGraphics
First Printing / First Edition April 2013

CONTENTS

Chapter 1 • Early Man Chasing a Meal

Early man had to conquer his food and environment. In the initial days of Earth man had a great and unique understanding about what he was and how his body operated.

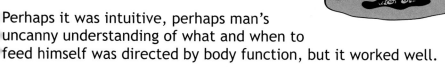

Perhaps it was intuitive, perhaps man's uncanny understanding of what and when to feed himself was directed by body function, but it worked well.

The body is well constructed like any good machine, yet our physiology includes a central computer (brain) and independent local intelligence centers making survival determinations in milliseconds.

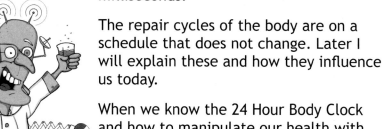

The repair cycles of the body are on a schedule that does not change. Later I will explain these and how they influence us today.

When we know the 24 Hour Body Clock and how to manipulate our health with this understanding, being healthy is easy.

Today the popular medical and nutritional powers have absolutely no idea what man needs based on their shoddy results and questionable products.

Modern Medicine grips the planet in a strangle hold, via their maniacal drugs and greed.

With use of brilliant double talk and chocking propaganda trumpeted by their media outlets, its blinding sales determination has paid off. They have amassed an empire almost incalculably vast.

A study performed by the Kaiser Foundation found that in 1980 Modern Medicine made 253 billion (US dollars) in sales. By expanding their drug definitions, by 1990 they made 714 billion (US dollars) in sales. Due to the FTC lifting bans on American TV advertising for drugs, they made a mind warping 2.3 TRILLION U.S. DOLLARS in sales. As of 2013 they are estimated to be over 2.7 trillion in skyrocketing sales income.

Because of Modern Medicine and Big Pharma's income needs, mankind is squarely in their crosshairs.

Governments share in the money accrued via yearly cash inflow from medication sales. Groups like the FDA require yearly Big Pharma payments for the privilege of selling to you and me.

What drives the modern mess that passes for nutrition and healing is a no holds barred run for income.

Factually, "obese" describes 2/3rds of the public in some localities, yet, obesity is 100% preventable. Uncontrolled eating and the problems it brings are such lucrative income streams; they will not be abandoned until the public is wise enough to stop partaking in them.

We do not catch disease; we buy it and eat it for breakfast, lunch and dinner. What we do to ourselves in the name of eating can be best described as self-poisoning and or self-torture.

Man's success beating the elements that early man struggled with has led him to such leisure time; his own welfare has become a game of chance.

Do people really live life like a game a chance? You know people who lust for the weekend and use as many mind and reality altering chemicals as they can afford.

The world is spoon fed a steady diet of "you are not responsible for the condition in which you find yourself." Believing this, we are likely to accept an invitation for lap-band surgery or a drug cocktail meant to suppress our body functions (like indigestion), ensuring worsening health.

Early man did not have the opportunity to reach into a refrigerator for food; he had to hunt it down. The man of the hour among those at camp was the hunter. His or her job was to feed the group or they starved.

Hunter Gatherers did all they could by gathering fruit, vegetables and hunting. Digging up roots and picking fruit was much easier than hunting animals that were fast, strong and might fight back.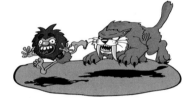

Many Anthropologists argue due to our less than canine teeth we are natural herbivores. That may be true but what defines man is a need for whole foods.

As we uncover the mystery that is man, we will siphon off the false data, conjecture and hearsay. With the flotsam and jetsam gone, it becomes very clear who we are, and what we need to do and eat to survive well.

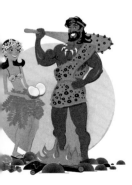

We can recapture our health thought gone long ago. The body never forgot how to be healthy, we just forgot the truth. The next 90 pages or so remembers what we forgot. The bridges are still there to be used if we hold and apply the truth.

The truth is here waiting for you to rediscover. I promise you can understand and use the gifts contained here. Let's find the "you" that you used to know, or may never knew existed.

Chapter 2 • **Life vs. Inner Toxicity**

Life ceases to exist if its cells are made to stand in their own waste. Organisms and cells immersed in such rubbish will subsequently reabsorb the junk. It is intense unforgiving contact. The body is not invincible, even slight association with man-made chemical garbage can cause illness. In the world of science they wrongly call this phenomenon "disease."

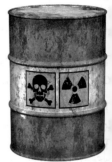

Opportunistic organism can exist in this waste, and even flourish. Without question, self-toxicity is highly erosive and eventually fatal to the cells from which it derives unless reduced or detoxed. These toxins are cancers.

We sanely fear environmental toxins, household cleaners, GMOs, junk food, preservatives and the Modern Medical toxins called medications. Our worst most destructive, other than strong poisons, pale to our self-generated toxic waste due to physical function, not supported, due to poisoning from a lousy diet. When our own lactic and uric acids linger in our body, i.e. muscles and joints, debilitating symptoms and illness await. The result is, we will have pain leading to physical breakdown.

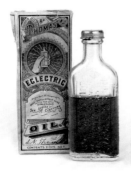

Toxins are always made of the same things; processed cellular waste acids not excreted or ingested alkalis. Be very clear there are no healthy alkalis if used in any volume as food, supplement or water.

The only purpose alkalis serve in the human body is for immune system activation when nothing else works. Alkalis are so toxic to human cells, if the body can't resist and remove them, they build and cause tumors.

In tiny amounts alkalis are used as an immune system activation device. Alkalis are what medications are made from. Simple herbals to complex chemotherapy, in the end are alkali in the makeup or action. Alkalis attack.

The body is systematically constructed to eliminate waste so life can advance and not be poisoned by its own waste.

The byproduct of cell metabolism is alkali waste. We already know cells do not flourish if they are standing in their own trash. The detoxification channels of the body were established just after fertilization to handle our internal cleansing job. As life grows, these channels never change.

The roots of the Liver and Kidneys sprang from the initial or 1st cell, as the body began to develop organs.

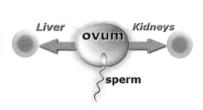

Every organ of the body uses channels of detoxification that were set at the time of conception. Growing, the inseminated ovum splits becoming 2 cells. The new cells become our liver and kidneys which hinge our detoxification system.

The Liver and Kidneys were built to hinge our detoxification network.

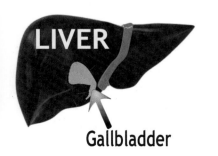

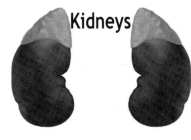

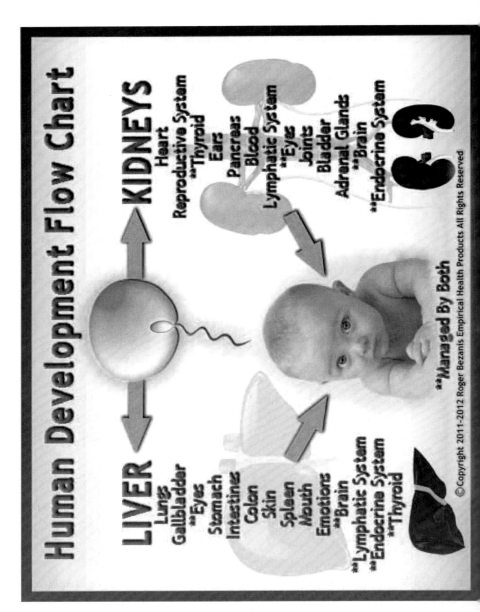

Human Development Flow Chart

KIDNEYS
Heart
Reproductive System
**Thyroid
Ears
Pancreas
Blood
Lymphatic System
**Eyes
Joints
Bladder
Adrenal Glands
**Brain
**Endocrine System

LIVER
Lungs
Gallbladder
**Eyes
Stomach
Intestines
Colon
Skin
Spleen
Mouth
Emotions
**Brain
**Lymphatic System
**Endocrine System
**Thyroid

**Managed By Both

Chapter 3 • Making Cellular Food

From our diet, our liver makes chemicals to be sent to our cells for energy creation. In the cells the chemicals are further processed like in a fireplace, releasing their energy potential. It is our Mitochondria that make our energy.

Mitochondria: *A structure in a living cell, in which biochemical processes of respiration and energy production occur.*

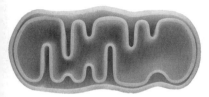 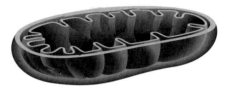

Above: A cross section of human Mitochondria, our cellular energy producers.

Looking at the structures above you may notice they are shaped a bit like the human intestinal tract. That is a correct assessment. When nature discovers a structure and function that works, it uses the mold over and over again.

The mitochondrion (plural of mitochondria), are like an assembly line producing energy in an orderly fashion. Once produced, energy is released for our use. Then the process starts again until the cell finally dies.

The final well known device mitochondrion are comparable to, is the common fireplace. Fuel goes in, energy is released.

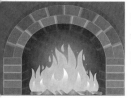

Regardless of what we call our intercellular power plants, they produce energy for life.

Human cells may have one or several mitochondrion making energy. If cells are defending the body by holding waste (like a jail cell), they are unable to make energy. Thus, mitochondria die. We will feel lethargic or exhausted. Keeping the body detoxed of waste is vital for our health.

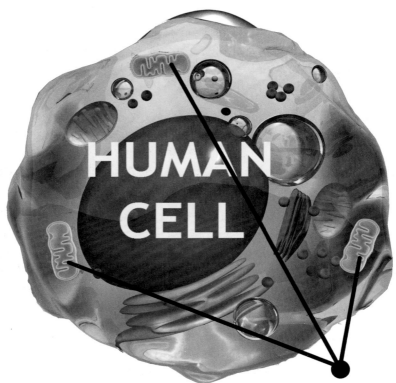

HUMAN CELL

Mitochondria

If you do not have fuel in your body, your body will strain and even fall asleep trying to make energy.

Chapter 4 • Chemicals and Life

Life pursues chemicals it needs and rejects those harming or slowing it down. The above may sound obvious yet mankind generally ignores this chasing tasty toxic chemicals. When irritating chemicals come in contact with human physiology, we are signaled via pain or a sensation declaring "warning."

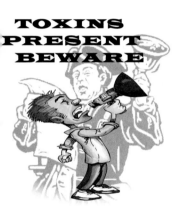

TOXINS PRESENT BEWARE

The kidneys and the liver are our town criers for the body. The majority of this job falls to the kidneys as they regulate much of the body.

If we have dogged pain, it is due to persistent toxic exposure. Pain is often mislabeled by Modern Medicine as disease yet as the body is detoxed free of waste, pain and illness vanish.

The old joke of seeing a doctor and telling him; "Every time I hit my head like this (bang) it hurts, what should I do?" Doctor; "Don't hit your head like that." It sounds simple yet, that is the message the body is giving us. The problem is we do not understand its language of pains and sensations.

Our body is a sentient entity which logically computes survival solutions to the most complicated obstacles man and this planet can create. Its maxim is to survive as long and as well as it is possible regardless of hindrance.

Long term survival is the target that drives our body. We on the other hand have knowingly or unknowingly made pursuing pleasure our goal.

The above outlines the great divide between what we want, verses what the body wants. These two goals are in conflict often.

Chapter 5 • **Body Verses Soul**

The trouble with man is he possesses the idea his body is indestructible. It is a fact, our soul or energy efficiently animates the body. But, the soul's indestructibleness is in direct conflict with the body's flesh and blood mortality. As the choice makers, our efforts good or bad can lengthen our lives or drastically speed our demise.

We can blame advertising or shortsightedness, but either way most of us run our body as if it is a nearly indestructible Volkswagen Bug or the AK47 (Russian assault rifle, legendary for its endurance and reliability).

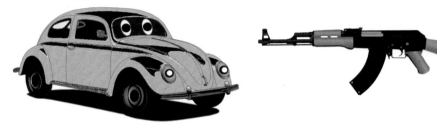

Perhaps we are trying to imbue our traits on our body. Regardless of why, our tug of war with our body is not winnable, as our body gets the last vote. When it is upset by poisons it tells us via pain and sensation.

Most ignore calls from their body to stop pouring in junk food and questionable "treats" as mankind's worsening conditions attests. The body clearly protests with pain or discomfort when it disagrees with our choices, yet many constantly use numbing medications hoping the problem will go away.

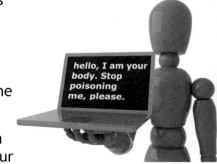

hello, I am your body. Stop poisoning me, please.

The only thing that goes away with regular use of pain medication is our health as these meds attack and eventually disables our immune system.

Acetaminophen is the leading pain medication worldwide. It is also the leading cause of chemical liver failure worldwide. Sad but true.

The use of pain killers and drugs in the body may seem sage and sometimes nothing else is strong enough to kill pain, yet their use should be brief and control returned to the body. Whatever chemicals we put into the body, the body must make sense of them and detox them out. While acetaminophen is an excellent pain blocker; it is even better at fully dismantling liver function. Regular use builds to liver cirrhosis or worse complete failure. Acetaminophen produces horrific damage.

The body is forced to endure what (we) its host pursues. If we want cupcakes we give it cupcakes. You may have noticed cupcake trees still do not grow anywhere on Earth.

Our misunderstanding of what food is and why we eat are lessons we have to relearn if we are to reverse the dwindling spiral of health on this planet.

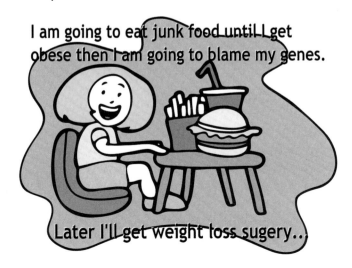

Chapter 6 • What the Words Mean

The development of language details our attitudes and habits at specific moments in time. Even long standing phrases tell us a story, such as "Breakfast is the most important meal of the day."

Our physiology is constructed to eat and run well on one or a maximum of two meals a day. Yet our eating habits have changed due to circumstance and the availability of food. Today, not having to hunt and compete for sustenance makes eating a rather leisurely experience.

- Not surprisingly the word dinner means: BREAK-THE-FAST

Language development illustrates dinner was the only meal man consistently ate. As dinner means Break-the-Fast, he ate it in the AM.

By eating 3 meals a day there is no fasting. It is of interest that the word obesity appears about 150 years after we started eating 2 meals a day with regularity.

- 800 BC Dinner is coined reflecting the universal morning meal
- 1500 AD Breakfast is coined, making dinner the evening meal.
- 1644-1650 AD Obesity enters our vocabulary.
- 1708-1812 Lunch is added as the midday meal.

The above data does not say man never ate more than one meal a day prior to the word Breakfast being coined. Language reflects customs and attitudes. When a word is invented it represents a change in behavior. The old accepted habits have transformed and the new habit has been adopted and is so named via the new word.

Without question the more frequently we eat the more the body is forced to deal with the extra energy, needed or not. In automotive terms, imagine an expandable gas tank that continually adjusts to fit the gas purchase habits of its driver. Due to this we have obesity.

Chapter 7 • **What is Food?**

Man's primary tussle with life involves two major obsessions; 1- Creating taste bud pleasing extreme tastes 2 – Altering his perceptions so he may experience a transformed version of reality to meet his moods and whims, via drugging.

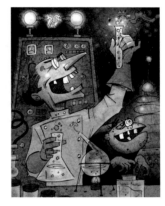

The above paragraph while simple outlines why man is preoccupied with medications / drugs. His pursuit of euphoria is now deforming and degrading his health.

As man toyed with fire and mixed this and that, he discovered a world of chemical cocktail brews. His senses thrilled, he built stronger solutions that fully blunted his awareness leaving him regularly numb. His eyesight began to fail, his hearing hollowed and his hands and feet stung with pins and needles, as he drifted into deeper chemical torment. Some call this Lupus or Fibromyalgia.

As a result, the plentiful gifts offered by Nature with their varying and healthy tastes seemed tame. Over time man has almost forgotten nature.

Presently some have never seen fresh fruit and vegetables. Instead man thinks food comes in boxes and cans or is frozen.

For the last 350 years man has been on a chemistry ride to oblivion. Obesity is now as high as 75% in some quarters; pre-adult hair loss is common in both sexes. Early or premature graying and menopause are now a pre-30's phenomena. What is the culprit of this turmoil?

The culprit in man's mutation is; his lust for chemicals that line a noose, he tied and placed around his neck. His wonderful noose now suffocates the life out of him.

Chapter 8 • **Introducing Fire**

It was a major success when prehistoric man discovered fire many millennia ago. With fire he could fight the cold and have light at night. The harnessing of fire changed man drastically as he could now employ torches to explore deep the dark. He could even live in a mountainside in places previously imagined to be dangerous with evil spirits.

He tried warming his food and discovered something happened to it, its `taste became more robust and the color of it intensified.

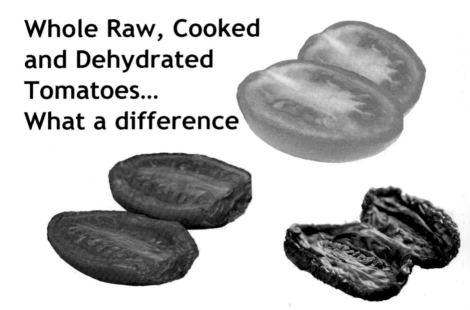

Whole Raw, Cooked and Dehydrated Tomatoes... What a difference

Nature uses red and orange as warning colors telling predators "no meal here." Bright colors tell us danger! Consult your memories, Red Ants (ouch), Black Widows with their red thorax symbol (poison), the yellow and orange Coral Snake, Wasps and Bees, etc. The message is clear, beware. The little RED Lady Bug? Even she is toxic to her predators.

The same warning nature gives us via bright colors transfers directly to our foods. In Nature, Whole Raw Foods are rich in color. Yet all chefs know, when they are cooked their colors deeply and robustly brighten.

What makes cooked foods appear so rich or deep? The heat from cooking changes their chemistry. As their enzymes (acids) shatter, it affects the surrounding food matter enhancing its color. Restaurants use this effect, as chefs' work hard to make their presentation burst with color.

Shattered enzymes are no longer viable for digesting food. They are essentially dead (denatured). Their colors become brighter as enzymes that gave life, oxidize changing their look. Regardless of what we call the final result, no cooked food enzyme is viable or able to support life. Cooking creates brightly colored former foods that warn us to stay away.

Cooked foods do not support life? That sounds harsh and it is, but it is nevertheless true.

Without active enzymes passing life into the future, life is dead. An apple seed carries a tiny enzyme that if planted can become an apple tree.

Life is lived via enzymes which are protein molecules. All life has them to a greater or lesser degree. Yet the same seed cooked first is denatured (dead) by the cooking, planted it will grow nothing.

Some claim nutrition is bolstered, strengthened or improved by cooking. The source of this insane idea is unknown. It seems to live in urban myth. Yet, no logic, testing or chemistry backs it up. But the saying justifies cooking and the sale of cookware and dehydrators.

Chapter 9 • **Cooking and The Nutrition Myth**

If cooking did improve nutrition we would climb into our oven and bake ourselves back to health. We would never get sunburns as burning would be therapeutic. Cooking fire would not kill.

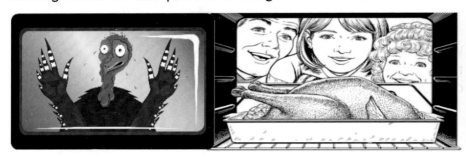

A tiny bit of logic goes a long way. The idea cooking improves nutrition is out of health nutrition left field, where it needs to be buried once and for all.

As seen via the tomato graphic (page 18), dehydrating and cooking cause the target of this abuse to shrink as fluids that are their lifeblood vanish.

Stating cooking improves nutrition is illogical. Cooking subtracts from what is cooked, it does not add something back.

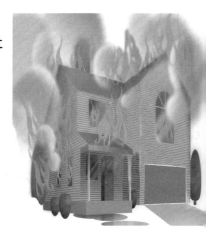

We can't burn down a house causing the house to replicate and become 3 or 4 or 5 to stand where one stood before. Fire does not multiply anything. It reduces what is on fire.

Fire destroys; it does not add or multiply.

When we burn a log in the fireplace:

Do we?:

A) Get more logs?

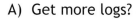

B) Get a pile of ash and no logs?

When energy is used up (enzymes are energy) waste is left behind that carries no easily usable energy. Here is the correct sequence of what happens when energy is used.

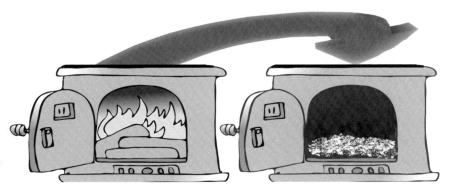

Burning logs do not start multiplying like a science fiction experiment. Fire burns away, it reduces, it shatters, but it does not enhance life.

Imagine if fire and cooking actually did improve what was cooked or set on fire. Fire would be like money. Arsonists would be rich artists and in high demand. In reality fire leaves waste behind not gold. Cooking leaves the wreckage of nutrition in its wake. A diet of 100% cooked food would kill most people in 90-180 days.

Everywhere in the universe physics apply. But to the inventor of the phrase "cooking improves nutrition" microscopic elements do not follow the laws of physics. To this individual cooking multiplies, it does not reduce.

You see the truth, but for others, old ideas die hard.

Let's look at lycopene (from tomatoes). Surely this is an exception! Lycopene pushers are rabid with their backward concepts. You know this is true as you have heard cooking releases more lycopene. If this is true, where does the additional lycopene come from? Was it hiding? Is it in a glass emergency container labeled "For More Lycopene Break Glass?"

An average tomato has .3 mgs lycopene. But cooked, many claim the same tomato has .6 mgs of lycopene. This is structurally impossible.

Does lycopene exist outside the world of physics? No, it reacts to heat just like every other nutrient in the universe. When a nutrient heats it shatters like a window hit with a rock.

Trying to be fair the amount of lycopene found in cooked tomatoes can appear to be greater than uncooked. Nutrients can seem to multiply when cooked because the lycopene molecules crumble. Cooking produces denatured useless parts of lycopene but no whole lycopene.

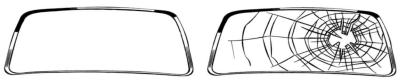

Once dead or denatured, no amount of hope or added chemicals reinvigorates dead cooked food elements. Again, 2 micrograms of lycopene or any enzyme do not increase in value via the cooking process. We lose healthful benefits of all food cooked, no exceptions.

Cooking has never, will never improve nutrition. Fire flatly destroys what it contacts. All reports to the contrary are nothing but ADVERTISING.

Man loves his cooking

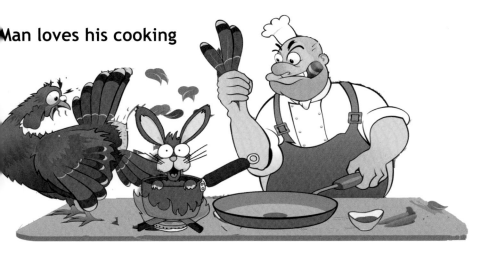

When man started cooking, he was amazed to feel warm from the inside. He soon discovered cooked food did not have the same characteristic as whole raw food. Its chemical content was denser and lacked nutrition while taking on medicinal qualities.

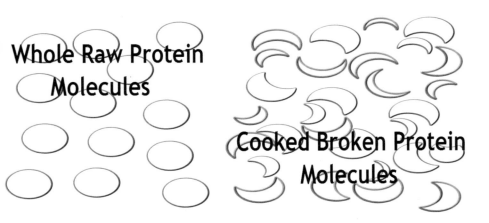

Whole Raw Protein Molecules

Cooked Broken Protein Molecules

Chapter 10 • **Food To Medicine**

The difference between Whole Raw Foods, Herbal Supplements, Homeopathy, Ayurveda, Medications / Drugs & extreme Chemotherapy is the density of their chemical makeup. Processing equals more density.

The major factor separating Whole Raw Foods from non-foods is; Whole foods are growing when found in nature. *What cannot grow and reproduce is dead or was never alive. Enzymes drive life*.

Foods are naturally acidic as enzymes are mild acidic protein molecules. Foods taken from Nature, if unaltered, are fully nutritional if eaten. Via enzyme action, real foods naturally decompose as they age.

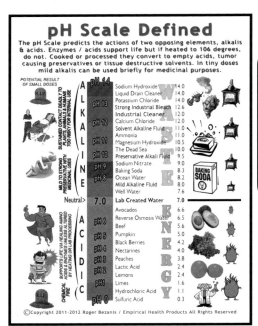

pH Scale Defined

The pH Scale predicts the actions of two opposing elements, alkalis & acids. Enzymes / acids support life but if heated to 106 degrees, do not. Cooked or processed they convert to empty acids, tumor causing preservatives or tissue destructive solvents. In tiny doses mild alkalis can be used briefly for medicinal purposes.

POTENTIAL RESULT OF SMALL DOSES

ALKALINE

SUSTAINED CONTACT DEADLY TO PLANTS, ANIMALS & HUMANS TOO RISKY FOR INTERNAL USE

MILD TO STRONG PRESERVATIVE WITH MEDICINAL USES

Sodium Hydroxide	14.0
Liquid Drain Cleaner	14.0
Potassium Chloride	14.0
Strong Industrial Bleach	12.6
Industrial Cleaner	12.0
Calcium Chloride	12.0
Solvent Alkaline Fluid	11.0
Ammonia	11.0
Magnesium Hydroxide	10.5
The Dead Sea	10.0
Preservative Alkali Fluid	9.5
Sodium Nitrate	9.0
Baking Soda	8.3
Ocean Water	8.2
Mild Alkaline Fluid	8.0
Well Water	7.6

Neutral> 7.0 Lab Created Water 7.0

ACIDIC

SUPPORTS LIFE VIA HEALING AMINO ACIDS & ENZYMES UNLESS ALTERED BY HEATING OR LAB PROCESSING

CHEMICAL FIRE

Avocados	6.6
Reverse Osmosis Water	6.5
Beef	5.6
Pumpkin	5.0
Black Berries	4.2
Nectarines	4.0
Peaches	3.8
Lactic Acid	2.4
Lemons	2.4
Limes	1.6
Hydrochloric Acid	1.1
Sulfuric Acid	0.3

WASTE ENERGY

©Copyright 2011-2012 Roger Bezanis / Empirical Health Products All Rights Reserved

The pH Scale is a life and death scale

Above 7.0 pH; no life exists, only harmful chemicals that dissolve cellular life or are preservative to cellular life stealing tumors. Tiny amounts of these chemicals can be used to awaken a sedated immune system to fight. Used this way they are called medicines, vitamins or supplements.

Below 6.9 pH is where life exists. The denser the protein content, the closer to 6.9 pH the food will be found. Fruit is light in protein and found lower on the scale. Fruit and vegetables are very healing to the body.

Food to be viable, support health and correct body function must be eaten in Whole Raw Form.

pH Scale Defined

The pH Scale predicts the actions of two opposing elements, alkalis & acids. Enzymes / acids support life but if heated to 106 degrees, do not. Cooked or processed they convert to empty acids, tumor causing preservatives or tissue destructive solvents. In tiny doses mild alkalis can be used briefly for medicinal purposes.

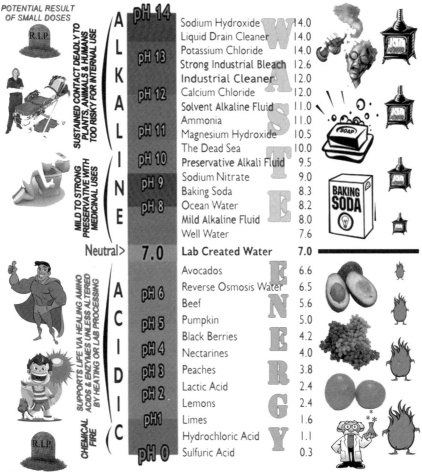

POTENTIAL RESULT OF SMALL DOSES

ALKALINE

SUSTAINED CONTACT DEADLY TO PLANTS, ANIMALS & HUMANS TOO RISKY FOR INTERNAL USE

MILD TO STRONG PRESERVATIVE WITH MEDICINAL USES

pH 14	Sodium Hydroxide	14.0
	Liquid Drain Cleaner	14.0
	Potassium Chloride	14.0
pH 13	Strong Industrial Bleach	12.6
	Industrial Cleaner	12.0
pH 12	Calcium Chloride	12.0
	Solvent Alkaline Fluid	11.0
	Ammonia	11.0
pH 11	Magnesium Hydroxide	10.5
	The Dead Sea	10.0
pH 10	Preservative Alkali Fluid	9.5
pH 9	Sodium Nitrate	9.0
	Baking Soda	8.3
pH 8	Ocean Water	8.2
	Mild Alkaline Fluid	8.0
	Well Water	7.6
Neutral> 7.0	**Lab Created Water**	7.0
	Avocados	6.6
pH 6	Reverse Osmosis Water	6.5
	Beef	5.6
pH 5	Pumpkin	5.0
	Black Berries	4.2
pH 4	Nectarines	4.0
pH 3	Peaches	3.8
pH 2	Lactic Acid	2.4
	Lemons	2.4
pH 1	Limes	1.6
	Hydrochloric Acid	1.1
pH 0	Sulfuric Acid	0.3

WASTE

ENERGY

ACIDIC

SUPPORTS LIFE VIA HEALING AMINO ACIDS & ENZYMES UNLESS ALTERED BY HEATING OR LAB PROCESSING

CHEMICAL FIRE

R.I.P.

SOAP

BAKING SODA

Mom's chicken soup factually was and is medicinal. A medicine is a condensed substance that was made in a lab, via heat and reduction, or cooked in a kitchen. When medicines are made at home on a stove, or in an oven, they are generally weaker than Big Pharma drugs, but are nonetheless medicinal by definition.

Many try to live on a cooked food diet with no food value. Some are only lucky enough to get a bite or two of something Raw and healthy per week. Sadly many adolescents are in severe nutritional danger. Due to this problem, today's parents are expected to out-live their children.

Unless we take responsibility for our own condition and state of health, each of us will get worse. Maintaining and correcting one's health with a Whole Food Raw Food diet can repair our worsening trends. Not doing so, we buy a ticket to a painful place where drugs and surgery are common.

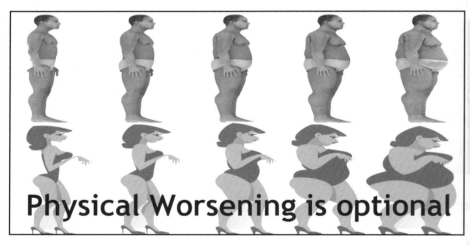

Physical Worsening is optional

Some only eat a piece of lettuce or tomato found in a sandwich, once a week or so. There are those who eat nothing but junk food. For them life is eventually painful as their body slowly devours its muscle, bone and usable fat for food. If seen by an MD they will be told they are diseased.

Man discovered the medicinal value of cooked food through trial and error. The medicinal value of roots, twigs, barks and flowers were discovered by watching sick animals graze. Factually anything we eat affects us and is healing or harmful depending on how much we consume.

The Father of Medicine Hippocrates, said; "let the food be your medicine and the medicine be your food." Preparation determines if food stays food or becomes medicine. It is all in the preparation.

Coca leaves are used in Columbian religious rites and creates a buzz when chewed. Because the leaves are so powerful, years of use can result in severe tooth decay and loss.

If one tried to overdose chewing coca leaves (which after processing becomes cocaine), the person would get sick and vomit long before they died.

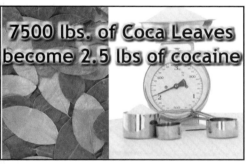

Even something as safe as water if consumed faster than the kidneys can filter it can be fatal. About 25 ounce (0.739 liters) can be filtered by healthy kidneys per hour.

Depending on stress via diet, drugs, activity and environment, we should drink between 80-120 ounces (2.36588 - 3.54882 liters) water a day. Sufficient water intake is critical for survival. For some, consuming a gallon of water a day will not be enough.

Only oxygen is more important than water. Do not drink Distilled or Alkaline water, as they have been made into drugs. To fully grasp the full subject of water, read my second book, "pH MADNESS."

The longer a substance is cooked, distilled or processed, the stronger the taste will be as its enzymes shatter becoming smaller, the substance will be thicker as cooking evaporates its water.

Raw Whole Foods are raw because their enzymes are whole, intact and uncooked. Whole raw enzyme rich foods from the earth have the potential to grow if planted. Raw foods left unattended rot as their enzymes cannibalize all available energy, until only dust remains.

When cooked food is left, over time it does not turn to dust, it dries to a solid chunk of something that was once food. Mummies are an example of what happens when flesh is dried out and preserved. The book "pH MADNESS" details this transformation.

Freezing food destroys its enzymes as the enzyme molecules burst when frozen, expanding by 8-9%.

Many mix fruit and veggies in a smoothie or raw mixed drink. This is problematic as enzymes attack each other making an inert mix. Just as gang member do not get along with police, enzymes are combative too.

In fruit and veggies mixes, even if the enzymes are the same pH, mixing them, they become a new substance or neutral (flat) mix.

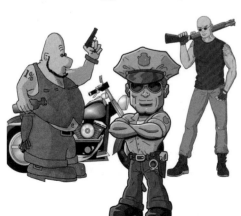

Mixing two items such as ice and warm water creates a new item, not warm or ice.

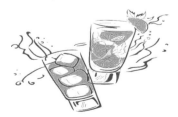

Chapter 11 • The Speed of Enzymes

Humans are inventors, which is a wonderful attribute but incredibly harmful when we consider that Nature cannot be reinvented. Such attempts have given us artificial orange juice (Tang & Sunny Delight) as well as Muscle Milk, which is not muscle or milk.

The difference between eating a salad versus drinking mixed juice or a smoothie is, once enzyme molecules are ruptured, there is no repair possible. Using after meal enzymes is folly.

A single fruit like orange juice has a few days of shelf life as its enzymes are not in combat with others. But it is healthiest if consumed within in minutes of squeezing.

As mentioned earlier mixed enzymes become combatants attacking each other aggressively trying to dissolve or digest what they encounter. Their purpose is to supply the power to release energy. Two opposing enzymes will attack each other as do acids and alkalis as per the pH Scale.

When acids compete, a surgery mix results that is essentially cooked dead food matter. Enzymatic cooking results when an acid rich enzyme solution such as orange juice is squeezed over beef or fish. The acid starts to cook or digest what it touches leaving meat that is chemically cooked.

Humans love to invent by cooking

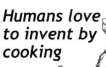

Enzymes LOVE to fight

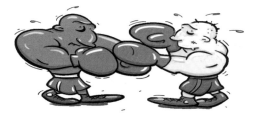

A common belief is that enzymes can be replaced after being destroyed by cooking. This is a complete fallacy. Believing enzymes can be brought back to life with post meal capsuled enzymes, assumes man can play God via chemistry. If you recall the novel and movie Frankenstein, you know it like replacing enzymes is science fiction too.

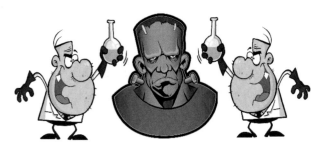

The fire of cooking always destroys what it touches otherwise we would not fear fire. Enzymatic cooking is just as efficient as fire, because enzymes are chemical fire.

The stomach uses a tiny bit of hydrochloric acid to start digesting our meals and to aid in killing parasites. When we consume layer upon layer of cooked food, the meals compost elongating digestive time by hours.

When we develop indigestion (heartburn, GIRD, Acid Reflux), the stomach is using the last remains of its hydrochloric acid attempting to ask for more acid not less. Advertising commonly tells us we have too much acid via indigestion. The truth is indigestion is caused by reduced stomach acid not too much.

Using enzymes after a meal, allows a worn stomach to resupply with acid, as cooked food has stretched its resources to the limit. Adding enzymes do not solve the problem, they just mask it.

The best way to heal indigestion is to NOT eat empty cooked foods that create the issue in the first place.

These foods are wonderful in healing indigestion and also aid the liver.

BIG 6 CITRUS SOURCES

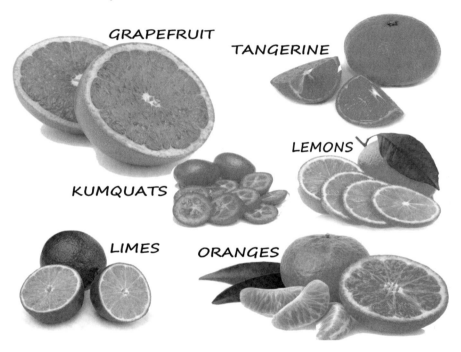

GRAPEFRUIT

TANGERINE

LEMONS

KUMQUATS

LIMES

ORANGES

Citrus is nearly magic in its ability to heal the liver, kill parasites, aid with digestion and repair indigestion.

If people knew how important the use of citrus is to the human body, they would have it in their kitchen every week for use daily.

Those doctors who warn against eating fruit if candida is present are lost, as citrus aids in the healing of troubling candida.

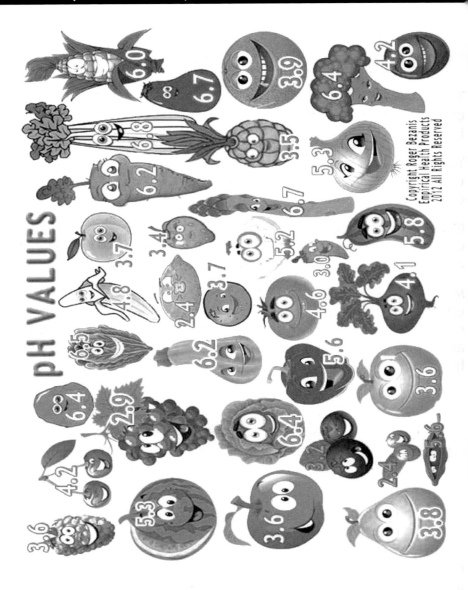

Humans can repair stomach acid and heal indigestion with use of citrus as it is very close (via pH) to the gut's hydrochloric acid. Tangerines, Limes, Oranges, Grapefruit, Lemons, Pomelos and Kumquats all are low in pH and rebuild Hydrochloric Acid.

Stomach Acid is 1.1 pH

Citrus is 1.9 to 2-4 pH

The two elements above are very close on the pH scale and derived directly from nature, unlike the cooked food that creates indigestion.

Yes, indigestion is an unnatural occurrence and only takes place if the body is made toxic due to poor processed meals, and or use of chemicals that block the stomach's ability to function.

If one has indigestion and cannot find a fresh tangerine or orange, even though vinegar is processed, it can be used to reset stomach acid.

Make no mistake the above paragraph is in no way endorsing the use of vinegar or any processed food for regular use. Vinegar like some cooked or processed foods can be used as mild medicinals, as they are more concentrated than herbals. Most cooked foods have no use.

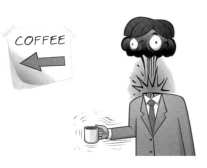

Coffee is now said to have medicinal qualities. This is an outrageous lie as caffeine offers 95-99% destruction to cells as it paves the way to tumor building and cancers body-wide. It is "the most widely used mind altering drug on Earth" as per the World Health Organization.

Caffeine is mankind's 3rd most popular toxin behind white sugar and salt. Yet, Big Coffee labors to hold on to its addicted public, as daily they are giving it up to pursue better health. (More caffeine on page 88)

Chapter 12 • Temperature, Life and Junk

The human body dies when its temperature reaches 106° (degrees) or 41.1c (Celsius). The reason for this is the subject of what makes raw food raw, namely enzymes. Enzymes survive at the same temperatures human life does as enzyme tendencies do not vary from one lifeform to the other. A good rule is never to do anything to your food that you would not survive such as cooking, freezing or blending, as enzymes are destroyed.

It is obvious that the more live and fresh our food is, the more nutritious it is to the body. It is even simpler than that. If food is not fresh and raw, it is either; decomposing (fermenting), dehydrated and therefore for intent and purposes nutritionally useless, or cooked "fully dead" food.

When life is gone it cannot be revived. When enzymes are gone but the former food remains, what we have is elegant looking vitamins. The trouble with vitamins is that they do not offer food value; they are only beneficial for digesting food if it is present. Vitamins do not feed life.

One fed vitamins but not food, will eventually succumb to starvation. Vitamins are equivalent to the keys to your car. Without keys your car will not run. But without your car the keys are useless. What is often ignored is that Whole Raw Fresh Food is packed with its own vitamins and needs no additional help. There is an INSANE argument that "the soil of the Earth is mineral depleted." This is totally as there is no fruit or vegetable growth without proper nutrients in the soil. The trouble with the soil is the polluted people eating from it not the soil.

If one briefly assessed a group of Whole Food Raw Foodists, they would rightly conclude, they are in amazing health. If the soil was depleted of minerals, Whole Food Raw Foodism would have vanished long ago like the dinosaurs. Instead RAW FOODS are healing bodies worldwide.

Junk food is enriched with vitamins and minerals because; if it was not, it would be so toxic it would create rapid discomfort on first bite.

Many people are so toxic that the mere taste of junk food immediately fosters warning symptoms, such as an urgent need to urinate, low back pain, blurry vision, moods and much more. The book Diagnostic Face Reading and Holistic Healing details every symptom the body can give and what organ the symptom is associated with. It is a must read as the symptoms lists are enormous and revealing.

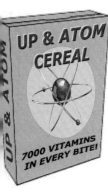

Mankind has a blind spot when comes to grains and cereal. Cereal is in no way "Whole or Raw Food," because of that it is without value. You may have noticed there are no cereal trees.

Steel cut oats are also processed. They are hulled and cut then blanched (cooked for a minimum of 30 seconds in boiling water) and packaged.

Cereal is a product served to fill a national need to feed the public inexpensively. Feeding the pubic filler does not equal nutrition. Full bellies may feel better bloated with milk soaked vitamin gushing cardboard. But the feeling is not nutritious. Oatmeal makes better wallpaper paste.

The use of grains was not an option for the Hunter Gatherer as his survival was a daily struggle. His ability to hunt kept his group going.

As man became more successful dominating and populating the land, he eventually congregated in villages and later cities. City living was free of day to day survival challenges known in the past. Man's new leisure created a population boom and a problem not foreseen, "how to feed everyone with the limited recourses available in the local country?"

Chapter 13 • **Digestive Evolution**

All life must at some time rest and repair itself. We know from earlier that the body logically evolved in stages hinged by its ability to rid itself of waste.

Body detoxification demands our cells remain free of waste or the body starts corroding. Our digestive survival is no different yet in many ways it is far more demanding. As the day progresses from morning, afternoon to evening, the job of digestive system repair becomes more and more critical.

Most people do not think about their body until something goes wrong. Then without training and full of false information, they see a doctor to make the pain go away.

The body is on an exact schedule and at no time does being drugged or ignored figure into the equation.

We must understand the body and allow it to perform its functions while honoring its repair schedule. If it is forced to postpone its scheduled repairs (you will see these later), it will not get a chance to execute them for another 24 hours.

Of course if we continually interrupt our body repair cycle by not going to bed, ingesting stimulants or eating late it will not be long until the body forces us to take heed of its needs, due to illness.

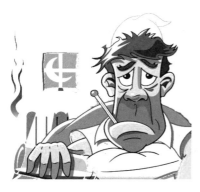

Advertising tells us we should eat when we want to and have whatever the heck we desire. It also tells us that if your body will not cooperate with your toxic cravings, you can silence it with a little purple pill.

When it comes to digestion, our habits make no sense.

Indigestion is a cry to change something, not ignore, sedate & re-pollute. Modern Medicine operates on the premise; "Life is best experienced through sedation." Not logical you say? Look at what is being sold, alcohol, sedatives, toxic pain remedies, indigestion blocking (sedating) formulas. Body sedation is wealth to Big Business.

The body is basically a machine while the digestive tract can be best described as a 9-5 shipping and receiving department. Our digestive tract is open 24 hours a day for emergencies, but if it is to operate at optimum levels it must be given time to perform vital repairs.

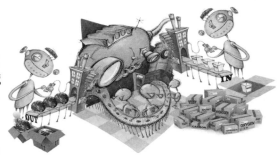

Imagine you ran a "shipping and receiving" department and:

- Receiving hours are 8 hours a day and 24 hours for emergencies
- It takes 4 hours to process a new package received
- Your workers need 10 hours of sleep to be able to function
- Your workers must go home at 5 pm to be fully rested
- No worker can go home until the last package received is shipped

Considering the previous five points, running your shipping department; when would you want your deliveries? Should they come in the morning or afternoon? Of course you would want your deliveries in the early AM.

Every business has business hours; our "imagined" shipping department opens at 9 AM and closes at 5 PM. As you will see, our digestive tract has almost the same hours of operation. Working late is a problem for both.

The analogy of the human digestive tract being much like a shipping and receiving department is a good one.

Both are or have to:
- Sort new deliveries
- Stressed by confusing deliveries
- Forced to store deliveries that take too long to sort (fat)
- Stressed by being forced to work overtime
- Need to eat, sleep and repair at night
- Ideally need to relax in the afternoon after a morning of work

Meals not digested in 24 hours become the beginnings of fat.

When we pick what we are going to eat, we are planning our future. Will the future be painful with arthritis like symptoms, sore muscle, creaky joints, poor sex drive, loss of hair, irritated skin, a weak heart, bad vision, vacillating moods, anger, short attention span, etc.?

Will our meal choices come at the right time during the day, so they can be digested & evacuated in 18-24 hours, ensuring a healthy mind and body?

For ideal health and to repair the body from past errors, we need to begin eating our meals at 9:00 AM & finish by 1:30 PM. This is based on the repair schedule of the digestive tract, seen in upcoming pages.

The shipping and receiving warehouse analogy is not just good, it is 100% accurate. If we eat late, the digestive tract is forced to work 24/7. Meal arrival and Digestion in the human body takes precedence over all other jobs. But it needs to rest and repair nightly or the body breaks down.

In a shipping department when deliveries arrive in the afternoon, it forces the crew to work overtime past normal closing time at 5 PM, as every package takes 4 hours to process. A package coming in at 3:30 PM means the guys can't leave until 7:30 PM, and there goes rest time and dinner. A delivery at 6:45 PM means the crew

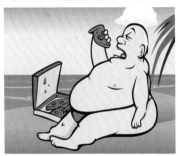

is working past midnight. The next day, the men are exhausted and dragging. Out of control package arrivals occurring daily; frustrates the crew and they start storing the parcels. As you have seen fat storage is nearly unlimited.

In the human body a frustrated digestive tract spells obesity.

The simpler and earlier we eat the better for digestion and healing.

Digestive Repair Times of the Digestive Tract

Intestines 5-7 AM (hydration 'water' is appropriate during this time)

Stomach 7-9 AM (this is why we should eat after 9 AM)

The Right Window To Eat is:

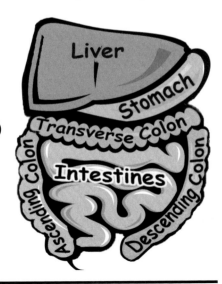

9 AM Until 1:30 PM

Ascending Colon 11 PM – 1 AM

Transverse Colon 1-3 AM

Descending Colon 3-5 AM

Intestines 5-7 AM (water okay)

Stomach 7-9 AM (eat after 9 AM)

Eating too late or too early is trouble.

How important is adhering to the right time to eat? If we ignore it and eat late the body will shut down to support digestive processes. This is why many fall asleep after a meal as the digestive tract steals all available energy.

What the last paragraph describes is a recipe' for heart attacks, strokes, leg cramps, brain fog, Lupus, Fibromyalgia, Chronic Fatigue, Crohn's, Wagner's, Hashimoto's, Epstein Barr, Mono, Osteoarthritis, Rheumatoid Arthritis, Arthritis, Post-Polio, Auto-Immune, Reynaud's, Shingles, Leaky Gut, Graves, Gilberts and even AIDs symptoms which can suddenly arise if the body is exposed to objectionable meals or wrong eating times.

All the "Disease Names" from the last paragraph have the same symptoms. What is behind this nightmare of diseases? Sales! Modern Medicine to be successful repackages and renames symptoms under fresh names to sell new medications. They do this to remain vital as a business that does not offer new products goes out of business.

Our worth at current estimation is 40 million US dollars for a life time of care. As this book is reprinted, add 1-2.5% a year for an approximation of our rising life time sickness value.

Again: The right window to eat is from 9 AM until 1:30 PM

Ascending Colon 11 PM - 1 AM

Transverse Colon 1-3 AM

Descending Colon 3-5 AM

Intestines 5-7 AM (water okay)

Stomach 7-9 AM (eat after 9 AM)

> Without use of stimulants it takes 7 -12½ hours for a meal to move from the mouth to the final stages of the Descending Colon. Therefore a meal eaten at 11 AM has just left the last stages of the Ascending Colon as it goes into its repair cycle.

The body runs on a 24 Hour Body Clock, our health is vital that we respect it.

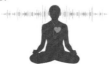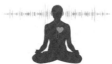

Every diet on the planet good or bad has one thing in common. They tell the user to not eat at night. Yet custom, habits, family unity and advertisers say the opposite.

I have been preaching against late meals since 2005 with the release of my book "Diagnostic Face Reading and Holistic Healing." Yet Asian Monks do not eat past 12 noon and the Black Foot Indians are early eaters as well.

Unlike my Monk and Black Foot Indian friends, I make a lot of noise and now even the anti-Natural Healing Crowd is moving in the right direction.

Researchers from Brigham and Women's Hospital in Boston and the University of Murcia studied 420 overweight people for 20-weeks in Spain. Dr. Frank Scheer, from BWH said: "This is the first large-scale prospective study to demonstrate that the timing of meals predicts weight-loss effectiveness. Our results indicate that late eaters displayed a slower weight-loss rate and lost significantly less weight than early eaters."

Late eaters also had lower estimated insulin sensitivity, a risk factor for diabetes.

The full story can be found in the Daily Mail Online, title: "It's not just what you eat, but when: *Eating lunch too late may make you fat." This was originally published in the "International Journal of Obesity"*

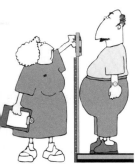

Let's pretend that you had not read the above or this earlier chapter explaining the function of the body via digestive repair times.

Let's only look at the idea of going to bed on a full stomach as eating dinner would dictate. Many of us eat because we are told to or because everyone else does. Many are brainwashed due to media and eat as their programing demands.

Like automatons many eat by the clock or due to the rumbling deep in their bellies. Body function is not taught effectively in schools and parents do their best repeating what they know or were told. This text is invaluable and must be passed on to anyone who will read these valuable lessons.

Ancient man heard rumblings in the caves and believing it was an upset God, made sacrifices to the cave. These sounds were rushing water or volcanic vent shafts belching.

Some people have been told abdominal rumbling is a call to feed the body. This belief not remedied spells obesity and physical decline in the long run. Stomach rumbling is not a bad thing.

The "rumble" or "growl" is sometimes heard as a normal part of digestion. It originates in the stomach or small intestines as muscles contract moving our meals forward with digestive juices down our 20- 30 feet of intestines and 5-8 feet of colon. An unhealthy intestinal tract may be as large as 40 feet in length. A diseased or unhealthy colon can be as long as 10 feet from start to finish.

The real name seldom used for "stomach growling" is borborygmus, pronounced, Bore-bore-rig-mus.

One starving without food for several days will hear borborygmus as air moves through the intestines. Most of us have never felt hunger so profound that the borborygmus they heard was a call to eat or die.

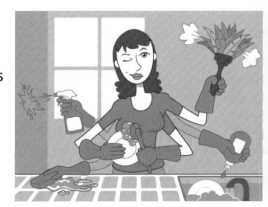

The digestive tract serves multiple functions from allowing for the extracting of nutriments to body "housecleaning."

The action of the intestines and colon that does the squeezing pushing our meals forward is called peristalsis, pronounced Par-ah-stall-sis.

The term peristalsis means the involuntary squeezing and relaxation of the muscles of the intestines or colon that allow earlier meals to move through the digestive tract.

Peristalsis creates the sound mentioned earlier called stomach growling or more precisely borborygmus (Bore-bore-rig-mus).

Unless we know the simple lessons of the above several paragraphs our own worry about what they mean can lead to our downfall.

Again diet logic has always said eating at night is harmful to the body stressing our vital organs. Mom's warnings about not going to bed on an empty stomach may have derived from "over mothering," or be a hold over passed down to us from relatives and movies remembering the Great Depression of 1929, when many starved.

Factually when one eats at night the body is so tormented that nightmares often ensue, the male prostate is weakened; diabetes (weak kidneys) is advanced and or created and much more including severe liver issues.

Organs attacked by evening eating include:

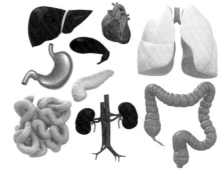

Liver	Kidneys
Heart	Colon
Lungs	Pancreas
Spleen	Gallbladder
Intestines	Adrenal
Glands	

Not to mention the male and female reproductive system.

Chapter 14 • The Successful Raw Food Diet

The body needs units of energy called food to enable it to perform biological functions; in support of a long term but impossible to achieve goal of surviving into infinity.

The biggest problem man has with his survival is the sandwiching of an immoral spirit or energy into a cellular lifeform needing regular sleep, hydration, feeding and care. The human body cannot run very fast, jump very high, fly without aid, walk through walls or on water, but here we are and this is our soup. The question is how to serve it logically.

We know from earlier chapters that food to be viable must be whole and raw. We know cooking interferes with and destroys nutrition as enzymes are cooked to death not able to withstand temperatures above 106° (degrees) or 41.1c (Celsius).

Life giving enzymes are acidic molecules of protein which compose all life yet, cooked they are worthless scrapes best used as filler.

We know digestion if fed healthy acids from fruit and veggies become alkali waste after our cell mitochondria makes energy out of these precious building blocks.

It is also known that some processed plants create acids that act like alkalis preserving what they touch and that these have mild medicinal values. And finally we know that medicines, supplements, herbals and all immune system activating substances are not foods, but mild to very strong alkalis that in enough volume will kill life.

The Road to Zero Nutrition Via Cooked Foods Can be Avoided by Eating Raw Foods

Eating Whole Raw Foods are the key to staying healthy. We do not want to eat ANY frozen, cooked, warmed, dehydrated, fermented, pickled, caned, flash pasteurized, High Pressure Pasteurized, dried, flaked, ground or mixed foods as their once viable enzymes are long gone.

We must be on guard not to be fooled by labels slyly listing "Fresh Squeezed" juice as "Never Heated" (HPP). The initials HPP stand for High Pressure Pasteurized. While HPP juice is never directly heated, the process applies 87,000 pounds of pressure per square inch of juice. The pressure creates heat due to the compression, as with pressure come's heat. This is a known physical law. Do not be fooled, High Pressure Pasteurize juice is heated and therefore dead and worthless.

Anyone understanding simple physics knows HPP advertising claims are pure untruths. Sadly more companies are switching to this process. Do not be hoodwinked by this deception as there is no life in HPP juices.

Super Foods are super advertising but there is no life found in a ground canister of such "foods." Ads for such products claim

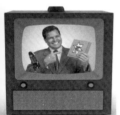

"improved nutrition" but there is none available in the mix. This can be proved by planting some in the ground and in good faith seeing what will grow. Factually, nothing grows if we plant a super food, not even mold.

Sprouting grains is a time consuming process but for those dedicated to the pursuit, it is growing and raw. But eat only the growing green stem not the seed. The seed is now empty as the growing stem now carries the nutritious life feeding enzymes we want.

There are no short cuts to life or nutrition.

There are basic laws we should know to stay healthy. A simple one is if it is new and improved; it did not come from Nature. New, Improved and Nature are incompatible.

The reasons to eat healthy should be as obvious as the reasons why we would not use cheap gasoline in our car. Performance will suffer. With the body we have a few more complex parts, but no replacement parts. When the body is unhappy it exhibits pain, soreness and stiffness. If these warnings are ignored long enough the body starts growing tumors, which if not detoxed out, accumulate to a point of suffocating the system. This is called cancer, which is completely avoidable and repairable via detoxification.

There are 3 ways to detoxify the body, they are; 1) Exercise as this forces cells to oxygenate and release waste. 2) Diet change, as this (if done right) frees the body from dietary toxic intake. This allows the safe release of stored toxins as the body begins repairing itself. 3) A full three month (or longer if necessary) detoxification program using various means such as herbals and formulas to aid the body in breaking down stored waste. A fourth way would be to combine any of the above three means.

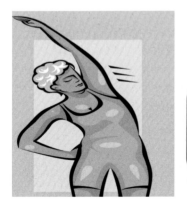 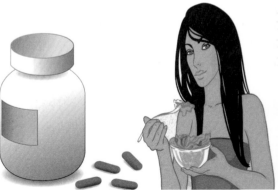

From the earlier chapters you already know the importance of respecting the body's rhythms. You know that meals should start at 9 AM and be finished by 1:30 PM. Eating Whole Raw Foods grown and taken from Nature, not altered by man, is also known factor. The rules that aid and heal the body are simple if we accept them and do not try to reinvent them.

Basic: Whole Food Raw Food Daily Plan:

The following plan can be used for a lifetime as it supplies the body with what it needs to keep it healthy and propel us back to better health.

I. Ideally awake at the same hour daily.

Waking at the same hour is vital as the body burns energy hourly and will weigh less an hour from now if you don't drink or eat anything. Waking at the same hour daily gives you an accurate measure of apples against apples.

II. Weigh yourself fully disrobed.

The reason why is so you can compare yesterday's weight to today measure with no added weight from clothes or underwire. This morning step also gives you valuable information telling you if you have gained or lost weight. Otherwise we are guessing via the fit of your clothes which is not accurate. If your weight is climbing or falling, and this is not your plan, you need to adjust the diet to your needs.

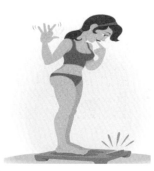 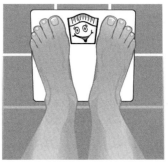 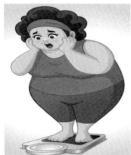

Weight is an accurate measure of meal digestion, it is not trivial data. The more you know about you, and how your body works the better commander of your health you will be. A victim is surprised by outcomes as they chose to not be involved in directing the actions that involved them. Another name for this is "victim." Using a scale daily at the same time every morning, sets the stage to make you a victor not a victim.

After rising, weighing and completing any other urgent bathroom routines, start hydrating as written in step A. below.

A. VITAL HYDRATION: Between 6-8:45 AM—HYDRATE! Drink10-24 ounces of Fresh Squeezed Orange, tangerine or grapefruit juice. Your ultimate target is to ingest 20-24 ounces of fresh squeezed over a 30 to 90 minute period prior to 9 AM. Do not make the mistake of gulping all of your juice down at once.

    Water Exception*: If you cannot get fresh squeezed juice, you can substitute equal amounts of REVERSE OSMOSIS WATER or SPRING WATER, (never drink alkaline water or distilled as they attack the body). Body hydration is vital to restarting your digestive tract in the mornings.*

    Your body has dehydrated during the previous night's sleep. The digestive tract is therefore stalled until you use hydration via water or fresh squeezed juice to turn the key and restart its engine.

FRESH SQUEEZED JUICE NOTE: *Fresh Squeezed means squeezed by hand or by a company that you know sells juice that was squeezed in the last 24 to 48 hours.*

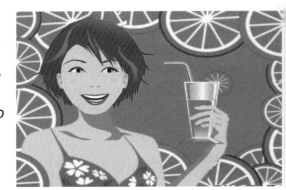

Patient NOTE: If any of the guidelines offered in this book, conflict with restrictions or protocols your doctor has previously given you, consult with him or her before following this book further.

MEAL #1 - BREAKFAST: The Day's 1ST and Main Meal

B. 9 AM BREAKFAST: This is your main meal of the day. Ideally, start your breakfast within a few minutes just before, at or just after 9 AM. This meal can be a large salad with ingredients from "BREAKFAST LIST" found in the "Raw Food Meal List." It can also be fruit as one chooses. See the "Fruit List" in the "Raw Food Meal List" too. To ancient man, this meal was sufficient to carry him (with some light fruit grazing) through the entire day.

The morning meal of breakfast should never be missed or avoided. If you cannot tolerate eating in the morning, do a detox for three months while you slowly ease foods into your morning habits and routines. The breakfast meal is the backbone of the day and the springboard to good health.

It may take 2 to 3 months to adjust to breakfast being your biggest meal. Until then, if lunch outsizes breakfast that is okay. Your goal is to eat your largest meal between 9 and 10 AM daily. Once this is habit you will wonder how you lived without this habits.

The word lunch is a tad under 300 years old. It developed due to commerce rather than need. Breakfast halls were used as town meeting halls at night. They started serving food and dinner was born.

Lunch also developed from a need for commerce. Why not serve a midday meal? It soon became popular and a tradition was created as well as the ground work for obesity.

PROTEIN NOTE: At any time during your breakfast, if you need dense protein, see the PROTEIN LIST and add some. Protein can be added to the lunch meal but it may slow digestion as it needs more time to breakdown. Heavy protein is best digested with the breakfast meal.

Protein Needs: Human protein needs have been reactionary since the 1973 American "Beef Shortage." This "crisis" was facilitated by Southern Corn Leaf Blight (SCLB- A fungus that destroyed corn) which caused the price of corn (livestock feed) to skyrocket. In turn livestock producers raised their prices by more than double in just days. Americans boycotted beef, shooting themselves in the foot as they refused to "have" what they wanted. When beef was finally available the supply had been cut by 75% and was nearly nonexistent. Suddenly we wanted something we could afford but couldn't find. Today we are still reeling from the 1973 beef shortage as its victims are now the old guard pushing their demented values on the rest of the planet. "Eat beef, the real food."

Factually we need perhaps 1/10th the protein content we consume on a daily basis. Vegetarians are living examples of this fact. If heavy protein content was crucial to life, dead vegetarians would be stacked like cords of wood along the side of the road.

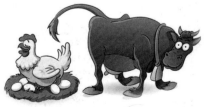

Today we bury ourselves in protein of every type. When we constantly crave more protein after eating a rich source, the source was without value and or so toxic via processing, the body cannot assimilate it.

MEAL #2 - LUNCH: *The Day's Final Meal*

C. <u>12 -1:30 LUNCH</u>: Lunch should be simpler than breakfast as we have so little time to digest it before the end of the day. It is best but not to eat foods that take extra time to digest. In the "Raw Food Meal Lists" I have included the "Digestive Challenging Foods" list, use it to build your meals. The best lunch foods are included in the LUNCH LIST, also in the Charts chapter.

Timing: We should be finished with lunch no later than 1:30 PM... Doing so supports the structure and function of the body and does not stress the digestive tract which controls the lion share of our energy. If we pass out after a meal, the meal was faulty.

SNACKS: Eating citrus (the whole fruit) after the morning meal aids with digestion, heals the liver, reactivates the digestive tract and much more. Citrus is one of Nature's amazingly adaptable foods that can be eaten all day long. Grapes are another dynamo food that alone heals the kidneys in all aspects.

DENSE PROTEIN NEEDS: If you have DENSE RAW PROTEIN NEEDS, see the protein list in the "Raw Food Meal Lists." Factually all Raw Foods contain protein as enzymes key their presence. The Dense Raw Protein List does not include all foods carrying protein, just some of the denser sources.

What is normal? Normal is run of the mill or the same as the group. If normal is ill, normal is abnormal. Using the Raw Food Diet ensures our best chance of being and or getting healthy.

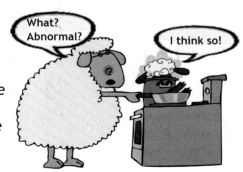

Intend yourself healthy and take the steps to make that happen. The Raw Food Diet works; make it your routine.

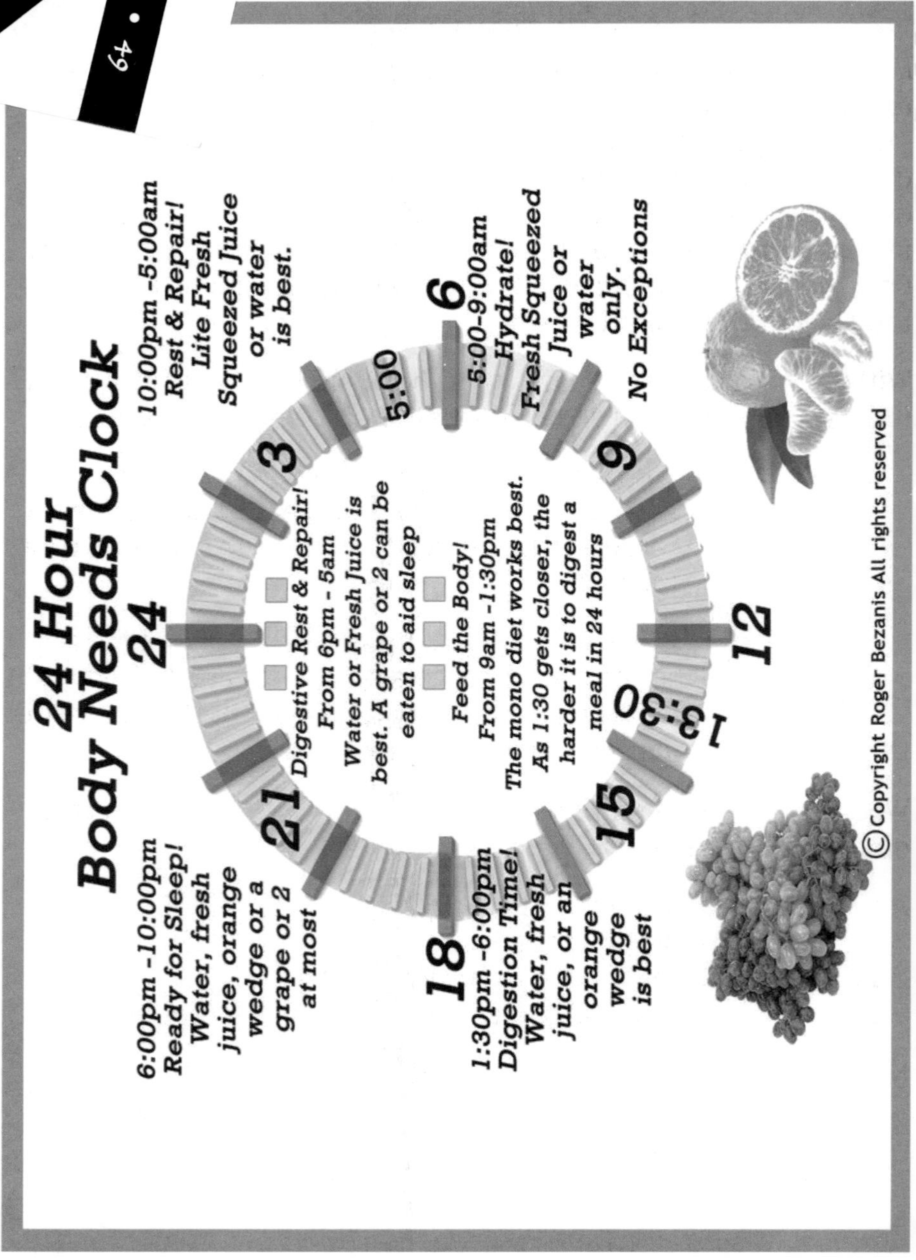
24 Hour
Body Needs Clock
24
3
5:00
6
9
12
13:30
15
18
21
10:00pm -5:00am
Rest & Repair!
Lite Fresh
Squeezed Juice
or water
is best.
5:00-9:00am
Hydrate!
Fresh Squeezed
Juice or
water
only.
No Exceptions
Digestive Rest & Repair!
From 6pm - 5am
Water or Fresh Juice is
best. A grape or 2 can be
eaten to aid sleep
Feed the Body!
From 9am -1:30pm
The mono diet works best.
As 1:30 gets closer, the
harder it is to digest a
meal in 24 hours
6:00pm -10:00pm
Ready for Sleep!
Water, fresh
juice, orange
wedge or a
grape or 2
at most
1:30pm -6:00pm
Digestion Time!
Water, fresh
juice, or an
orange
wedge
is best
© Copyright Roger Bezanis All rights reserved

Chapter 15 • The Mono Diet

Mono means singular or one. The Mono Diet is defined exclusively eating one food at a meal versus any kind of mixing. This is the purest form of meal eating we can incorporate into our diet. This approach is so easy on the body it is practically a non-event to eat a meal. Normal meals of mixed foods stress the body in every way as each food needs a different digestive treatment. Of course eating Whole Raw Foods eliminates most of this issue, the Mono Diet is even less stressful.

Without question the simplicity of the Mono Diet is as infallible as it gets. The mono diet is like a vacation for the digestive tract.

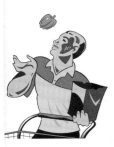

It is akin to juggling with one ball. In other words you are throwing a ball in the air and catching it. Throwing the same ball in the air and catching it, and so on.

There is no limit to how long the Mono Diet can be used as its success speaks for itself. Animals in the wild generally follow the Mono Diet as part of their habits. Humans adopted variety.

What can be eaten on the Mono Diet can vary from meal to meal or can stay the same all day long.

A successful example of the Mono Diet:
1. Breakfast (9 AM) 8 tangerines
2. Lunch (12 Noon) half a large cluster of grapes
3. Light nibbling of easily digested fruit or veggies until 3 PM.

Next Day:
1. Breakfast - Repeat
2. Lunch – Repeat
3. Light nibbling – Repeat

Following Day:
1. Breakfast - Repeat
2. Lunch – Repeat
3. Light nibbling - Repeat

Again, the Mono Diet works and can be repeated indefinitely with healthy WHOLE RAW FOODS.

The uses for the Mono Diet are endless. The foods eaten on the Mono Diet of course should be Raw, Whole and taken directly from Nature as no one ever sees a lion stand up at a kill and shout "Elk? Again! I want tofu!"

When one walks with Nature the body gets in sync and energizes to heal the worst conditions. Eating Whole Raw Foods is like getting a body guard to protect you. That is how powerful the gifts of Nature are to the human body.

The fruit or veggies chosen for meals during Mono Diet; can be pulled from the Breakfast, Lunch or Snack Lists, found in the Chart Chapter later in this book.

If we want to attack what MDs call disease from Fibromyalgia to Lupus and beyond, we are the beneficiary based on our discipline. The hallmark of this plan takes the most discipline. Nothing is more supportive to the body when it comes to eating.

The Mono Diet is so therapeutic it may not have limits as it unleashes the body's potential to heal via no outside interference. We can change our physical condition.

The same lists for Breakfast, Lunch and Snacks can be used to pick the item we will eat for our meal choice. This is the Raw Food Diet essentially made simpler.

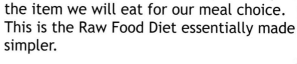

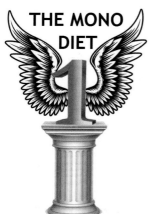

The Mono Diet makes healing possible and simple. As we already know the deception and complexity of Modern Medicine, drives us further into the muck. Think simple.

Be sure to eat enough to be satisfied as what you are eating, easily digests. Remember, we are juggling 1 ball. The Mono Diet works.

Chapter 16 • The False Raw Food Diet

Raw Foodists are not all the same. Some are Whole Food Raw Foodists, seen as extremists or purest by most. The leaders are the adoptees of the Mono Diet and The Raw Food Diet who apply and use the 24 Hour Body Clock written in the previous chapters.

Since Raw Foodism was purposed, it has been attacked to destroy the movement. A "crusade" to Whole Raw Foodism absolutely rocks and sinks the profits of the trillion dollar cooked food industry. We are surrounded by cooking. To not cook is near heresy.

Adoption of Raw Foodism threatens to dismantle the home kitchen as we know it. No Raw Foodist needs an oven and only needs a stove once in a blue moon to make homemade medicine. I will speak to Homemade Medicine later in the book.

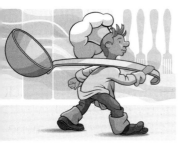

Pseudo Raw Foodists not only eat Whole Raw Foods, they eat frozen food, dehydrated food, Raw Pizza; Raw Pizza?

Grinding is very acceptable to some, as their only criteria to calling a creation Raw is; "did it start Raw" & "Is it cooked."

Raw means uncooked and unchanged by man. Yet to a False Raw Food eater, attaching the word "Raw" to a mixture is perfectly fine, opening the door to all manner of non-raw creativity.

What is Non-Raw Creativity? A mix called Super Food falls under this label as its contents are ground to flakes or powder. Nothing in "Super Food" canisters have the capacity to grow if planted.

"Super Food" and "Raw Food Bars" are a joke as they lack anything raw. There are no Raw Cereal trees or Raw Food Bar Trees; these are a dietary and marketing abomination.

Don't be fooled. Nothing labeled RAW is ever "Raw." Raw, means "Raw."

Picking a piece of fruit and eating it is as basic as raw gets. That is really eating "Raw." What makes this book and its approach so drastically different are the applications and alignment of Raw Foods, Food Digestive Times and body function awareness. Earlier texts such as the "80-10-10 diet" focus on building muscle without understanding body function as aligned with Earth's and our 24 Hour Body Clock.

Ignoring our 24 Hour Body Clock is like trying to ignore gravity. Good luck with eating anytime of the night or day and expecting the body to fall in line behind our impossible and slavish demands.

We possess all the pieces we need to understand and heal the body, we already have this data, but other books on the subject failed to connect the dots.

The "80-10-10 Diet" had most of the pieces yet completely missed on the times to eat and the body's repair cycle as obviously influenced by the Earth's and or own "24 Hour Clock."

Atkins & the Zone missed completely not understanding the body has needs based on Whole "Raw" Foods not just the remains of fats and proteins.

The Paleo Diet has some aspects correct regarding raw foods but, again has not a clue about our inner body clock affecting us. Paleo is good but negates the planet we live on ignoring its influence on our lives.

Knowing when to eat is as vital as what to eat. Out of sequence we get poor or limited results. The wrong sequence in eating is as backward as reversing the sequence in bowling by throwing pins at bowling balls.

The universe follows Natural Laws that ensure uniformity and a continuum of existence as we know it. We know that water douses fire, that gravity causes attraction to Earth and prevents us from jumping very high.

A vast list could be made of Natural Laws, but that is not the purpose of this tome.

Because the body is so well constructed and works so hard to compensate for our idiotic behavior, we forget it has needs. Factually most of us have no clue it has any needs at all, and just shovel in the junk. The term "Raw" is all the rage today. "Raw" will remain a buzzword long into the future as salesmen use it to secure your cash. Raw is not a Buzzword, it is a state of being. It is not a label.

No diet is as exacting and demanding as the Ancient Raw Food Diet and no diet can do what it does, which is; allow the body to rebalance itself.

Remember, any job done in the wrong sequence will create something other than what was intended. While the body appears to survive our diet faux pas, it slowly (or rapidly), gets worse by the day.

Doing The Ancient Raw Food Diet (TARFD), do TARFD, not some watered down version of it. The results come from following the correct sequence.

Not what you see below...

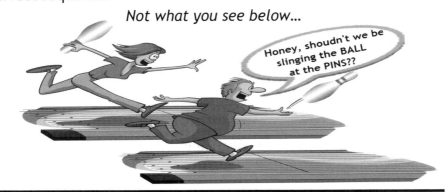

Honey, shoudn't we be slinging the BALL at the PINS??

Chapter 17 • **What About Meat Protein**

Whole Food Raw Foodism is based solely on getting all the enzymes and not allowing anything to be cooked or warmed. Athletes and enthusiasts have little compunction with eating Raw Meat too.

Eating Raw Meat has a long history and shows up in many cultures from Asia, Europe, the Middle East, Africa and the America's.

> *(From page 50)*
> *Factually we need perhaps 1/10 the protein content we consume on a daily basis. Vegetarians are living examples of this fact. If heavy protein content was crucial to life, dead vegetarians would be stacked like cords of wood along the side of the road.*

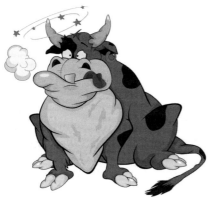

There are many passionate arguments for not eating meat protein of any type. These arguments are all valid from spiritual, moral, Earth conserving and body saving. Like it or not, cattle, fish and all game are exposed to and absorb the waste man makes to power and dominate the asteroid he calls home.

Beef is so costly to consume it is shocking cattle farmers can make a living. It takes enough water to float a destroyer to produce a marketable steer for slaughter.

Fish are so contaminated they are now continually found exhibiting both male and female reproductive organs, dual heads, multiple eyes and more.

For those determined to make raw meats and or fish part of their Ancient Raw Food Diet, despite health risks due to toxins, read on. As you know consuming meat is not only costly to our planet we risk our health due to hormone and chemical sludge found in its flesh.

Beware, raw meats are so dense in protein, a little goes a very long way.

Whereas other diet plans stress eating meat protein, it is due to few fanatics still reacting to the beef shortage of the early 1970's. Literally protein heavy diets fight a war long over. Due to this, vegetarians make up the smallest eating group on Earth today as meat obsession continues to rise.

Earlier chapters cover our decent into meat gorging due to historic events.

Beware; eating too much protein stresses the kidney creating protein spillage into the urine called Ketosis.

Body builders can follow the usual TARDF plan, with these additions:

With Breakfast Add:

- 1-3 thumb size pieces of Whole Raw Stew Beef

OR

- A thumb size to a palm size piece of Whole Raw Salmon or Tuna

With Lunch Add:

- Same as above

Chewing, it is important to chew fully before swallowing all beef, or little nutrition is garnered from it.

Chewing is important no matter what you are chewing as we have no additional teeth in the body after we swallow our meal bites. Remember poor chewing guarantees poor nutrition and eventual poor health.

It can take 5 minutes of dedicated chewing to release all of the enzymes available in a single piece of beef. If you are in a hurry to eat a piece of beef, it is better to pass and eat it later.

For those determined to consume meat protein as part of their routine, the above is how it is done.

What about eggs you ask? Eggs are the only dairy product that is not in some way processed and is therefore raw if eaten prior to cooking.

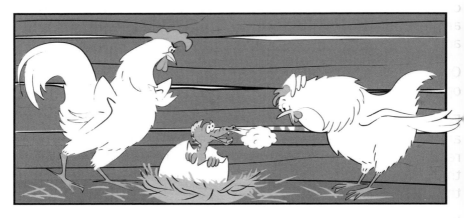

Cheese is mankind created; milk does not grow up and become an udder or a cow. Yogurt is no better than any other dairy product, even mixed with a few lactobacillus cultures. Yogurt at best is 70% bad and 30% good as it is in a dairy carrier. Yogurt is NOT raw, it is created.

An egg can potentially become a chic. By this rule alone, eggs are the only dairy product that is growing and therefore can be considered Raw.

A large egg carries 6 grams of protein. Factually unless one is continually tearing and rebuilding muscle via heavy workouts we do not need this much protein in 3 days.

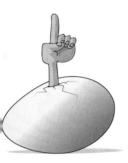

A near magic aid that goes unused by many protein loaders is magnesium as it is at the base of muscle function and building. Be sure to include it in your daily routine if you are a gym rat, body builder or athlete of any kind.

Raw Eggs get bad press due to salmonella which is blamed at every turn to keep people from using Raw Foods to improve them.

Factually big business will always strike out and try to destroy its competition (real or imagined) at every turn. Salmonella scares are just another avenue to this end. Be your own judge and jury and you win.

One who is responsible for himself and knows how his body operates is not privy to hoaxes and charades that keep us in fear.

Eggs can be eaten straight from the shell for those so inclined but are most often mixed and quickly consumed in orange juice. The reason you should quickly drink the frothy mix down, is because the two enzymes are acting against each other every moment they are mixed.

If the last line of the previous paragraph reminds you of the Mono Diet, it should, as it speaks directly to mixing enzymes.

To excel at anything from accounting to athletics we need to pay attention. If your stools become dense, hard, odiferous or liquid, they are unhealthy. Too much protein makes for very dense stools.

Beware and use a colon formula as needed or cut back on your protein intake.

When it comes to oil humanity is obsessed with the stuff. We love to smear it on our skin, cook with it, burn it, buy and sell it and eat it. In supplement form we seem to love it.

Oil continues to be valuable as we use it to power the industrial complex. The problem with oil is that the body cannot assimilate the goo.

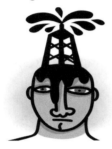

Using oil IN or ON the body is; clogs it fouling its operation. The only things that break down oil are strong acids which the body does not possess beyond the stomach and fire which the body does no generate. As you know, this book is about RAW FOODS. Not only is oil in no way Raw, it cannot be used or metabolized by the body. Oil can only be utilized by the body, it the body extracts it itself, from Whole Raw Foods. Oil supplements and topical uses must be avoided or we intoxicate the immune system with breakdown resistant sludge. As a protein source it is lousy unless eating it unaltered in whole raw foods.

Oil of any type including olive, soy, Omega 3 & 6, avocado, walnut; clogs the liver, disabling the immune system for hours. This is so well known, Hepatologists (liver doctors) the world over recognize and agree; oil must not be ingested or used on the skin.

Nuts are a huge source of oil and concentrated protein. The problem with them is that even raw nuts are quickly boiled before they are packaged as raw. If you have a personal connection with a Nut Farmer, then you can trust that the nuts you purchase are actually Raw.

Cashews in Nature are found in pods encased in toxic gel. Before they can be sold the gel is boiled off and then boiled again. Cashews labeled "raw" or not raw at all. Nuts are such a concentrated form of protein, they overwhelm the kidneys creating ketosis (kidney poisoning). Because of Botulism prevention rules, raw nuts are not commercially sold.

Chapter 18 • **Pesticides**

As you have discovered via this book, using Mother Nature to feed your body's needs is not only smart it is life giving and healing. As man drifts away from his roots in Nature, his life gets complicated to say the least.

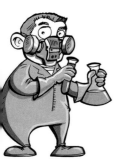

Organic produce is the best way to consume Raw Fruit and Veggies, yet it is a fact that in many parts of the world, they are hard to find. What should we do? Do we give up and eat gram crackers? No, the thing to do is reduce our risk as much as possible while we demand safe produce.

We should also realize that a few pesticides while not optimum, is far better than consuming a diet of cooked foods. As we know cooking creates intense concentrated concoctions that corrode and form tumors.

It is better to consume our Fruit and Veggies with pesticides while we demand their removal, than not eating Fruit and Veggies at all. The old adage, "The squeaky wheel gets the oil" still hold true. He who makes enough noise eventually is heard and wins.

Don't stand for GMO's or pesticides. You will be heard.

Until you have a better choice, get a good veggie wash and clean your fruit and veggies as much as possible prior to eating them.

Homemade Fruit and Veggie Wash

- 8 oz of Water
- 8 oz of Vinegar
- 2 tables spoons of Baking Soda

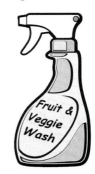

Mix for one minute in a blender to reduce the froth so it can be used in a spray bottle. The juice of 2 lemons can be added to the mix as a cleaning bonus.

Chapter 19 • **HCG Diet**

The HCG Diet like all other extremist diets has a limited shelf life of use before it stops producing results for one reason or the other.

HCG stands for Human Chorionic Gonadotropin. It is hormone that occurs naturally during pregnancy. Its purpose is to ready the body to carry a new life. Its presence sends the body of men and women into a pregnancy detoxification cycle. Yes, it sends both males and females into a pregnancy detoxification cycle. This causes the body to shed weight.

As it activates the entire system fooling it into action, it is used for low sperm count to counter the effects of a toxic lifestyle and infertility in women. The correct solution is not to fool the body but detox it free of waste.

The problem with the HCG diet is not its workability, as it does work when its guidelines are followed. The issue is that it is using a chemical (hormone) to fool the body into action.

As you know, Whole Food Raw Foodism is against the use of any chemicals unless used in an emergency as they alter our chemistry and function from head to toe. Medications are as subtle as a sledgehammer.

The HCG Diet has some use if it is used for a short time as per the instructions. The fact is unless the poor diet that caused the excess weight is changed, months after the HCG Diet is finished, the weight will be back. Then the person is in the Fat Soup again.

It is because of issues like what are mentioned above, that make the Ancient Raw Food Diet so necessary and workable. It not only can be used for a short time, it can be used for a lifetime.

Chapter 20 • Vegans & Vegetarians, Honey & Milk

There is absolutely nothing wrong with being a Vegan or Vegetarian until the individual starts cooking their nutrients away.

Cooking destroys our nutrients rendering our food nothing but a plate of vitamins. For all intents and purposes, that is the most we can expect after cooking food. Factually the nutrition we get from food is lost upon cooking. A slight alteration with heat destroys the life in food forever.

Many have an idea that breads, pasta and all manner of processed junk is okay as long as it is not derived from or contain any meat or dairy products.

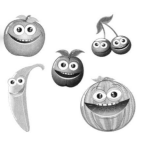

A life lived within the guidelines above leads to all manner of abuse. Candy and sweets have no business in the Ancient Raw Food Diet of any program to heal the body.

If food needs to be sweetened to be palatable the eater needs to detox him or herself free of waste. One craves what they are most toxic to and unless we are detoxed as well as possible, odd cravings will arise from time to time.

Is there a safe sweetener or suggested sweetener to use as a Whole Food Raw Foodist? No, as no sweetener other than freshly squeezed juice is whole and raw. The option to sweeten with orange juice or other citrus or fresh squeezed pineapple juice is open. But ask yourself why?

Once one is "Whole and Raw," foods burst with flavor. As for vegans and vegetarians, those that apply the Ancient Raw Food Diet with their current passion and drive will have great success.

Vegans and Vegetarians should be the healthiest people on Earth. With the Ancient Raw Food Diet it is a reality.

Arguing over definitions separates most groups, Raw Foodist are no different. The term Raw means:

- Not altered by man beyond chopping or juicing
- It was growing in Nature on a plant or in the Earth
- It is a fleshy part of an aquatic or land animal

What separates food from former food, are enzymes that are the keys to life. In the proper structure (a living entity plant or animal) enzymes are what animates the entity and allows it to reproduce. Once gone there is no way to replace them.

Honey is often argued to be Raw. It is not. Honey is best described as BEE REGURGITATION. The bee ingests pollen which mixes with fluid in its "crop" (bee stomach). Then it is regurgitated to be re-eaten. This process is repeated until the pollen is an aqueous solution in the drone bee's crop. Finally it is spit up again to air dry. Honey is best used medicinally.

Milk is another enigma that people love to argue about. Milk is often considered Raw but when we really look at it, it is not.

Milk is a fluid not unlike blood. Its sole purpose is to feed a growing calf for 8-12 months. Cow's milk like any lactation fluid is not meant to feed a species for a lifetime. It certainly is not meant to be used interspecies.

One might logically question why Humans would drink cow's milk as it is from an animal species completely unlike man. Many cynically ask why we don't warehouse human mothers to milk them dry for general consumption. Milking human lacto-slaves would be disgusting and inhumane. Odd because harvesting cows for bovine vampire abuse causes bleeding utters, and that is normal, sane and nutritious.

A living Raw Food is defined by its ability to reproduce and exist as a species. Milk is in no way a species, it is the fluid of life for a calf or goat. People can try to argue this but they are arguing from passion not logic.

A side note: Almond and Soy milk are as "Live and Raw" as a corpse. At one time almonds and soy beans were raw, but processing them destroyed them leaving the remains of their enzymes in their wake.

A good test of a Raw Food is; does it have the capacity to reproduce if planted in the ground, or is it as a species, like a fish. If the former is true and it has not been destroyed via processing or cooking, it is a Whole Raw Food.

Part of what drives people to ingest milk is tradition, as cattle's herding in the Americas was a huge livelihood for many. When money is involved obsession results.

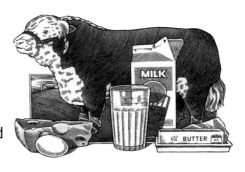

Yet the milking of cows occurred as early as 6000 years ago according to some scientists.

The fact is all humans are lactose intolerant, yet the irritation varies from one individual to another. Some argue that man developed a genetic mutation that allowed him to ingest milk between 5000-4000 BC.

What actually happened was; due to regular ingestion, human bodies stopped offering warning symptoms of toxicity due to wayward milk consumption. In the end milk is consumed out of habit causing a myriad of issues from loose stools to constipation, high cholesterol and more.

Avoid it or fall victim to this non-raw food trap.

The evidence is overwhelming. Milk is reprehensibly riddled with pesticides, hormones and much more. No Whole Food Raw Foodist would ever consume milk, cheese, butter or yogurt. These products are so bad; especially milk it must be loudly admonished for being such a toxic chemical cocktail of dangers.

The dairy industry is given vast latitude in what they feed and inject dairy cattle to increase milk yield. A sampling of milk yields the traces of various pain killers, growth hormones, antibiotics and even anti-inflammatory medications.

Science spouts; "These are trace elements and not enough to do harm." The cumulative effect over time is unmistakable as girls are reaching puberty as early as 8 years old. Astonishingly 40 years ago, the average woman was B cup (breast). In 2010 the average size topped a C!

Baldness in men under 20 is now common. In some places obesity tops 75%. This is happening because we are bathing our cells in a chemical cocktail allowed by our governments. Everyday meats produce and more are GMO'd.

As per the University of Spain, here is some of what is found in milk...

Niflumic	Florfenicol	Funixin
Acid Mefenamic	Estone	Pyrimethamine
Acid Ketoprofen	17B-estradiol	Diclofenac
Diclofenac	17a-ethinylestadiol	Triclosan
Phenylbutazone	Naproxen	

The list above features anti-inflammatory drugs, painkillers and hormones. White spots under your nails are a telltale sign of these. If we get ill we see an MD and they win.

Chapter 21 • Fasting, Juicing and Moderation

Fasting is the time honored method of detoxing the body through pure absence of all food for as long as 45 days. It is the most rigorous form of detoxification there is as the body is forced to devour its fat for food.

Because fat is a depository for toxins missed by liver processing, breaking it down can be painful. As our fat breaks down we may feel a headache, dizzy, tipsy and more depending on what is stored in the fat. We may think we are free from our past chemical transgressions, yet a small portion of these travel with us into the future.

Fasting has been practiced since biblical times and of course before that. The two most important elements to survival on Earth are Air and Water. Extreme but limited fasting is done for a day or two with no water at all and of course the complete absence of food. This type of fasting is extremely stressful and is not recommended.

The better our digestion the healthier we are. The better the food we eat the better our digestion and the healthier we are again. One leads right to the other. The Ancient Raw Food Diet (TARFD), is the most effective eating program there is as it receives no resistance from the body.

Weight Gain is a simple process of not expelling all of our meal in a 24 hour time. Just a few ounces a day if not expelled leads to huge weight gain yearly.

.5 oz of food not expelled daily x 365 days = 11.41 lbs yearly

1 oz of food not expelled daily x 365 days = 22.81 lbs yearly

2 oz of food not expelled daily x 365 days = 45.63 lbs yearly

3 oz of food not expelled daily x 365 days = 68.44 lbs yearly

Fasting can be done a variety of different was as long as meal restriction is part of the equation. The Master Cleanse or Lemonade diet is very popular and works famously. Below I present a popular variation that has worked with great success. It should be done for no more than 45 days.

Citrus Flush Fast Mix (PART 1)

In a ½ gallon jug (64 ounces) combine the following with Reverse Osmosis or Spring Water:

The juice from one lemon
The juice from 4 oranges or tangerines
1 teaspoon of garlic juice
3 teaspoons of dark "Grade B" maple syrup
1-5 teaspoons of cayenne pepper (to taste)
1-3 teaspoons to cinnamon powder (to taste)

- Drink the above Citrus Flush Fast Mix over the course of a day.
- Use another 64 ounce jug to ingest additional water daily as needed. This water should also be Reverse Osmosis or Spring Water.
- Your combined fluid intake including Citrus Flush mix and water should between 80 to 128 ounces per day.
- The Citrus Flush Fast Mix bottle must be empty by 7:00 PM.

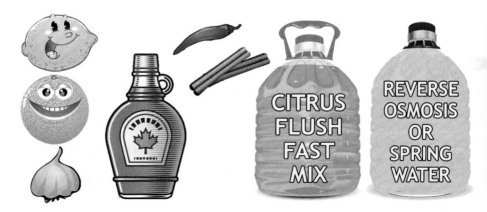

Citrus Flush Fast Mix (PART 2)

It is vital to the Citrus Flush Fast to start every morning with a bowel flush. The reason for this is because there are no solid meals moving through your intestines or colon after the second or third day of your fast.

With nothing to push waste now being excreted from our cells, the bowel will reabsorb them and we become very toxic. Flushing bowel is vital for a fast to work successfully.

This is where the Sea Salt Flush is used. This is the option offered below.

Sea Salt Bowel Flush (final step of the Citrus Fast)
It is very important to schedule this flush at least an hour prior to all of your commitments that would preclude your quick use of a toilet. You are about to embark on a tremendous flush of the bowel.

In a 32 ounce bottle mix:

- Two level teaspoons of Sea Salt
- 32 ounces of warm water Spring or Reverse Osmosis Water
- Shake well until the Sea Salt appears to be dissolved
- Drink down the solution in 20 minutes
- Stay next to a toilet as the Sea Salt is a Cathartic

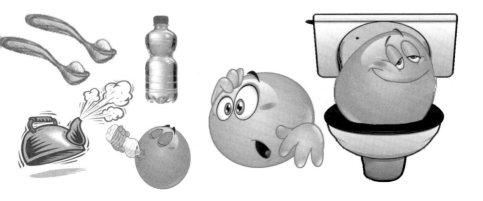

Citrus Flush Fast Mix (PART 3)

As you can see by the last page, the corning bowel flush after each day of the Citrus Flush Fast is vital or we can become backed up and very uncomfortable. Of course being very close to restroom facilities are important too as the body completely rejects the salt water as it races out.

For those who want to forgo using Sea Salt there are two options.

A. You can use a powerful Herbal Colon Formula (of your choosing) to flushing out your bowels throughout the day.

B. You can also substitute Purple or White Grape Juice (not frozen) as these act as a bowel purge as well.

Colon Formula Flushing
Using a powerful herbal formula, make sure your bowels are emptying at least once a day if not 3 times for the first 2-4 days.

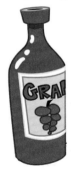

Grape Juice Bowel Purging
Purchase grape juice in a glass bottle, as this is the purest form, as plastic can leach into the juice.

How much you will need to purge your bowel will vary from person to person. Some will have great results with 8-16 ounces in the morning while others will need 32 ounces. Nursing a bottle of grape juice all day long does not produce the same purging result for most.

Regardless of how much you need to use to purge your bowel, it is best to drink your grape juice as early as possible. No, you cannot substitute wine!

Some will do a Grape Juice Fast for 30 to 45 days. Beware, purging can occur rapidly. Many describe the "grape juice stool," as being dark green or purple with a distinct odor of grape juice. Do not be surprised when it comes. No, grape juice is NOT raw, it is being used as a medicinal.

Juicing

Juicing is a favorite way many have for getting all of their fruit and veggies in a day. There is an issue that must be discussed as we look at the popular subject.

Logically, mixing raw juices makes loads of sense right? Not so fast, when two competing enzymes are mixed as mentioned in the chapter "What is Food," we end up with a new solution that is neither one nor the other.

Not only that, the new mixture is losing enzymes by the second as the enzymes are battling to stay alive.

If you choose to Juice fruit, I strongly suggest you juice one fruit and drink it at a time.

If you are so inclined to test this for yourself, by all means do so. But, if you do, I again urge you to; drink your juice mix in no more than 3 minutes as time is life when enzymes are mixed.

Some will do a juice fast like a grape juice fast for weeks. Depending on the person it may be done for 35 days or longer as the body is getting nutrition.

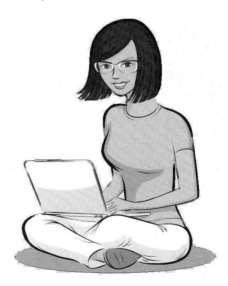

Stacy Brown fasted on tangerines for 45 days with fantastic results. She drank 60-90 ounces of water a day and kept her bowel moving with an herbal colon formula. Weight came off, skin became soft and supple and her moods and energy were fantastic.

Moderation

We have all read and heard "a little won't hurt you," or "moderation is the spice of life." These statements derive from those selling poisons. As business needs customers they will do nearly anything to hold onto market share. The worst thing that can happen to a business is a loss of customers and therefore business.

As a result, the idea of moderation was concocted during the 15th century (1400-1499 AD) to ensure people did not change their habits drastically.

Many "love" to preach moderation, as if it's a lost book of the bible. Because moderation seems so soothing and logical, people hold it close. Those same folks (some very ill) annoyingly chirp this odd word as a right and a privilege to continue to get physically worse.

Moderation always involves bad habits that addiction demands the addicted not change. The businesses selling the addictions, laugh all the way to the bank.

Factually a little poison is still poison. Now consider what moderation really is, in action:

Go ahead have a little:

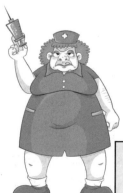

- White sugar
- Salt
- Coffee
- Bread
- Butter
- Pizza
- Hot Dogs

- Beer
- Cereal
- Soy
- Cooked food

- Junk Food
- Chocolate
- Wine

Moderation invites slow death... How nice...

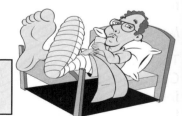

Chapter 22 • Crimes Against the Sea Today

There is a belief that government are in the business of protecting its public. Perhaps that derives from when we were very small. We remember mom, dad, sister, brother, etc., would act as our protector. We were buffered against the evils of the world, against worries and danger because we were shrouded in a protective glow. We were warned in advance of danger with "Don't touch that!"

Did we expect this blanket of security would last forever?

There is time worn evidence; governments have little interest in protecting its "all" of its people. To be minority was a ticket to abuse in Poland, France, Germany, Austria and the rest of Europe at the start of WWII.

Today for enough money the world's governments will sell out their publics in the faint hope it will go unnoticed, or not be too messy.

Where is our keeper, the keeper that watched over us? The job fell to each of us. If we are not doing the chore, it is not getting done.

Governments protect those who invest in them. When it comes to receiving privileges, money speaks loudly. When the money in question is trillions, billions or even a puny few millions in dollars, it gets attention, a lot of attention.

Government surveys prove sea dumped pollutants cause birth defects and cancers and much more. Why does the dumping continue?

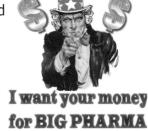

Money talks...

The world we live in is lined in cash. Governments are not out for our best interests, they're out for the best deal from those who pay them.

I want your money for BIG PHARMA

Lobbyists make deals around the world with gifts and payoffs supplied to them by their backers. For this "exchange" they buy excellent treatment for their employers. The gifts are delivered by 3rd parties to ensure the gifts are hard to trace back.

Even investigators are bought which causes any inquiry to linger, be dropped or name the guilty party, a young man in the mailroom.

Make no mistake Big Brother government is doing something to protect the public. They are enforcing that small warning labels are added to the packaging of fish that are known to be toxic.

How nice. When seafood should be banned, the sea labeled toxic, and the oceans cleaned up, we get small warning labels.

Shrimp in the Gulf are mutating: From Al Jazeera- Siggs of malignant impact on the regional ecosystem are ominous: horribly mutated shrimp, fish with oozing sores, underdeveloped blue crabs lacking claws, eyeless crabs and shrimp. "Disturbingly, not only do the shrimp lack eyes, they even lack eye sockets."

It is not in the best interest of Government to bite the hand of the hand that feeds you. British Petroleum as let off the hook.

"We also seeing eyeless fish, and fish lacking even eye-sockets, and fish with lesions, fish without covers over their gills, others with large pink masses hanging off their eyes and gills."

The Gulf of Mexico needs to be dredged clean. But we get warning labels...

Are all fish everywhere on Earth toxic?

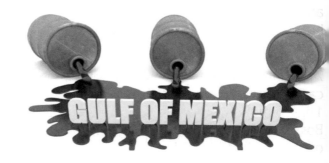

No, all the fish on earth are not toxic with chemicals. If they were raised in a small pond under strict controls with no pesticides, they would be safe. Pond raised fish makeup less that 1% of all fish on the planet.

In 2010 Portsmouth University scientists became aware of fish consistently infected with the psychotropic drug Prozac. The innocent are becoming riddled with psych meds simply by eating fish. If they are commercially caught, there is nothing one can do but abstain.

The seafood industry is a billion dollar business. Jan 14, 2009: A 2-headed bass was found in the Noosa River in Australia.

You know Australia, (The Land Down Under) where men are men and water is clean...

This is not an indictment of Australia or Australians; it is a question of "What have we as mankind done to ourselves?"

26 June 2012 (Portland, Maine) Owner, Bill Sarro's seafood shop and restaurant took possession of 100 pounds of lobsters. Normal lobsters are greenish brown. Sarro's shipment contained 6 bright orange crustaceans. Getting just 1 off color lobster is a rare occurrence. The odds of finding 6, in 100 pounds; is beyond calculation.

Another dealer (New Meadows Lobster in Portland, Maine) discovered 3 freakish lobsters; 1 bright orange, 1 bright blue and 1 calico lobster. White, pink, red and black lobsters have been found in 2012.

The odds? Finding a blue lobster is 1-in-2 million; orange is 1-in-10 million. Yellow & orange-and-black calico lobsters are pegged at 1-in-30 million, split colored are 1-in-50 million, amazingly, a split color lobster was found in Boston in October 2012. Finally the white lobsters are the rarest of all at 1-in-100 million.

Lobsters are sea bottom dwellers; the same ocean bottom where chemicals from hair dye, to pharmaceutical drug discard settles.

We do not live in a bubble things do affects us. When we mindlessly attack nature we are attacking ourselves. Most would agree, chemical companies, the oil cartel and more are guilty of crimes against humanity for their daily dumping of sewage.

From the Potomac Conservancy: The Potomac Conservancy, which focuses its interests on Washington D.C's biggest river, recently called for new research to help them figure out why male smallmouth bass in the Potomac are beginning to carry underdeveloped eggs in their testes.

"More than 80% of the male bass fish in Washington's major river are now exhibiting female traits such as egg production because of a "toxic stew" of pollutants," reports The Guardian. "Intersex fish probably result from drugs, such as the contraceptive pill, and other chemicals being flushed into the water and have been found right across the US."

From the US Geological Survey: Mercury has been well known as an environmental pollutant for several decades. As early as the 1950¹s it was established that emissions of mercury to the environment could have serious effects on human health.

These early studies demonstrated that fish and other wildlife from various ecosystems commonly attain mercury levels of toxicological concern when directly affected by mercury-containing emissions from human-related activities. Human health concerns arise when fish and wildlife from these ecosystems are consumed by humans.

During the past decade, a new trend has emerged with regard to mercury pollution. Investigations initiated in the late 1980's in the northern states of the U.S., Canada, and Nordic countries found that fish, mainly from nutrient-poor lakes and often in very remote areas, commonly have high levels of mercury.

More recent fish sampling surveys in other regions of the U.S. have shown widespread mercury contamination in streams, wetlands, reservoirs, and lakes. To date, 33 states have issued fish consumption advisories because of mercury contamination.

Today we are waste deep in toxins from every angle. What we dump in our water ways, we like to pretend it disappears as the oceans are so vast. It does not, in 2008 actor Jeremy Piven was hospitalized for mercury poisoning. He had been eating tuna sushi 5 days a week.

As the toxicity in our oceans and waterways grow we are told to eat fish once a week.

From the -The **Department of Health: <u>Question</u>:** "Should I stop eating fish?" **<u>Answer</u>:** "No! Fish is good and part of a healthy diet, so don't stop eating fish!"

A 1995 study from the American Public Health Association: The EPA reports that "Literally every American has accumulated measurable levels of 30 various toxic compounds that linger in their adipose (fat) tissue."

A newer report claims that 157 toxins are now found in fatty tissue.

We could call breast milk "Pesticide Milk" as it features lindane (gamma-bhc), chlordane, dieldrin (causing convulsions, coughing, dizziness, headaches, nausea, weakness, tremors and more), dioxins and 65 isomers of PCBs.

Routinely 35 types of PCB's are passed along in male semen. The human body has become a spongy toxic waste repository. These chemicals unleash a cornucopia of dangers on the bodies of both sexes. Every day the population at large is victimized by these silent killers.

These toxins are coming to us via sea and inland fishing. Toxic life altering toxins that we humans dump in our waterways are more than a threat. Yet we're told to eat fish once a week. The reason why we are told to consume fish at all is money.

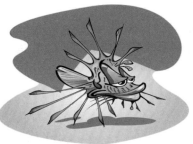

Even though eating fish today is akin to slow suicide, those recommending that we eat fish are free men. How is this possible? Because the criminals making the statements; also make the laws.

Can we eat fish? Of course we can eat fish. We can also drink battery acid, play in traffic & skydive without a parachute.

Toxins are created by lab technicians, given to industry then dumped in the oceans for safe keeping. This is akin to sweeping dirt into your Christmas turkey and serving it. Once in the waters many chemicals settle on the ocean floor before they work their way back up the food chain and into our bellies.

These toxins infect planktons which are eaten by filter feeders. Larger fish eat the filter feeders, which are eaten by larger fish, which are caught in nets and fed to the public.

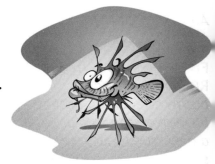

In many parts of the US more than 70% of male fish species are found displaying dual sexual organs.

Toxic accumulations from seafood cause metal based toxins to short circuit the body causing all manner of trouble including heart attacks. This can include mutations.

On the CDC (Center for Disease Control) website they endorse: >>>Dietary Guidelines for Americans, a healthy eating plan<<<:
- Emphasizes fruits, vegetables, whole grains, and fat-free or low-fat milk and milk products
- Includes lean meats, poultry, FISH, beans, eggs, and nuts
- Is low in saturated fats, trans fats, cholesterol, salt (sodium), added sugars and stays within your daily calorie needs

MUTATED FISH FOUND IN AUSTRALIA *An inquiry into the discovery of two-headed fish at a Noosa River hatchery has found proof the deformities were caused by agricultural chemicals, according to media reports.*

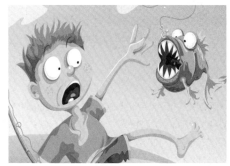

Inquiry taskforce member, Dr Matt Landos has been reported as saying the report, due to be released soon, would show the mutations found at Sunland Fish Hatchery created by a toxic cocktail including carbendazim, nonylphenol, beta-cyfluthrin, methidathion, trichlorfon, methoxyfenozide, atrazine and endosulfan.

All (of the above chemicals) are approved individually for use in Australia.

From <u>Discover News</u>: MORE HERMAPHRODITE FISH IN U.S. RIVERS *Male fish with female anatomy are appearing in river basins across the United States. Male fish with female body parts have been showing up in our nation's rivers for a while now, but a new study that found a surprising number of mixed-up fish may shed new light on ecosystem health.*

From the Mississippi to the Rio Grande, from the Appalachia to the Colorado, researchers found large numbers of river fish with egg cells in their testes, particularly in two species: smallmouth and largemouth bass.

At some sites, more than 70 percent of males from these species were intersex, a condition that has been linked to lowered sperm production, trouble reproducing and other negative health consequences.

Male largemouth bass and smallmouth bass with female anatomy are showing up in river basins across the United States. At some sites, as much as 91 percent of local, male largemouth bass are intersex.

In the Pee Dee River at Bucksport, S.C., for example, 91 percent of male largemouth bass had female parts, along with 60 percent of males in the Apalachicola River at Blountstown, Fla., and 50 percent in the Savannah River at two sites in Georgia.

More than 65 percent of male smallmouth bass were intersex in parts of Minnesota, Idaho and Colorado.

If fish started knocking on our doors telling us they are too polluted for human consumption perhaps that would help.

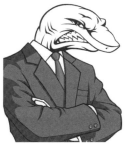

(CNN) -- The world's appetite for fish is now at an al- time high according to the United Nations. Figures from the U.N.'s Food & Agriculture Organization (FAO) states fish is currently the most-traded food commodity, worth around $102 billion in 2008.

As per CNN, in 2007, humans consumed 37 pounds of fish per person. At that rate, we will continue advancing into obesity, diabetes (irritated kidneys), tumors and debilitation. Today degenerative physical issues are found at the end of fishing lines, thus we are toxic seas of pollution.

From the **World Health Organization (WHO)**: Worldwide, about a billion people rely on fish as their main source of animal proteins.

Dependence on fish is usually higher in coastal than in inland areas. About 20% of the world's population derives at least one-fifth of its animal protein intake from fish, and some small island states depend almost exclusively on fish.

From **Green Facts**: In 2010 the average human ate 36.08 lbs (16.4 kg) of fish. The Chinese per capita eat 57.42 pounds of fish (26.4 kg)! Thanks to this toxic intake they are fast becoming one of the most toxic people on the planet. With this kind of rabid fish consumption and their building love affair with Western Junk Food, it won't be long until they fully embrace Western Medicine and its poisons.

Big Pharma is waiting patiently in the wings to help the Chinese when they cry uncle.

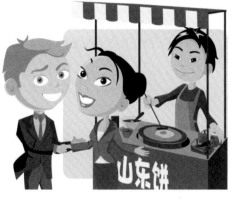

Fish are deadly almost everywhere unless we harvest them in our own back yard, in our own pond. Then we would have to let any current toxicity in the fish breed itself out over time. In 2 years we could safely eat our backyard fish. Otherwise the steady flow of hazardous toxins entering rivers & seas from urban sewerage & industrial discharge makes eating fish unsafe.

How is big brother protecting us? They are gallantly doing it with small warning labels. Sorry we were past warning labels in the 1970's. A total ban on fish is what is called for.

Yet there is no ban on fish from the CDC just advice to include it in our diet. How thoughtful.

We have all been told that mankind is destroying the planet, yet it is still here. We are told that we are killing the planet for our kids. Yet we really haven't changed. Here is a slightly different point of view.

1) If we believe in past and future lives, we are destroying the planet for ourselves in the future.

2) If we are God fearing folk with Heaven in mind we are destroying the planet for our offspring and current mankind. Incidentally, by the way and just in passing, how do you think God feels about our actions polluting his creation?

3) If we are atheists, then our conscious is our guide. If we are carefree and atheist we care little about our actions. If we are atheist but "fellow man minded" we care deeply.

It doesn't matter what our religious beliefs are or if we have them at all. We must be responsible for our actions good and bad.

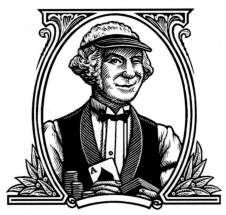

Each of us must make a decision as to who runs our lives. It is up to us to make decisions based on sound information. The information contained in the above paragraphs and pages is loud and clear.

The governments of the world care little what we do as long as it is legal and they get paid. For us, currently it is a gamble to eat any aquatic life.

The solution to today's land and sea damage will take 400 years to repair. Presently to safely eat fish, we must grow them ourselves, and not harvest any for at 7 seven generations or risk toxicity. Selling home fish hatcheries will be the new business soon enough. Until then, never eat fish unless you have grown them yourself.

Chapter 23 • The Final Step Detoxification

Detoxification is vital as the human body is basically a sponge. To aid the liver and the body from being made ill, cells capture and hold toxins.

The idea of Free Radicals is science fiction. Free Radical; is a term that has been with us since the early 1900's. It simply means toxin. That is all a Free Radical is, it is just a toxin. Please substitute Toxin for Free Radical, thus putting it on the junk heap of confusing terms.

Another invented term with us since the early 1900's is Antioxidant. This just means immune system supportive either by being a free standing vitamin or an enzyme rich nutrient. Antioxidant is a poorly constructed word for its present use, as it means anti-oxidize or preserve. The last thing any lifeform should have contact with is a preservative; to do so is death to the infected cell.

The comingling of Antioxidants and Free Radicals occurred at the Alexis Park Hotel in 1993, in Las Vegas at the 1st "Anti-Aging Convention." I know this, as I was there as a vendor with my herbal formulas. None of us had a clue about "Anti-Aging." It was a sales pitch thought up by marketers trying to make a buck. It opened a Pandora's Box of confusion.

Cells that do not age are best described as cancerous. Beware of anyone selling you anything that oxidizes your cells or has a high Oxidative Reduction Potential (ORP). If the product actually works (such as Alkaline Water which preserves cells), it causes cancer. This type of product used for any length of time; deranges our cells and can kill the user.

Detoxification should be done once or twice a year, for 3 months. Today the toxic load is so great, a once a year detox may not be enough. All switching to Whole Food Raw Foods, your diet detoxes you. For you, a good detox is in order when you first start, but if you remain toxin free, you may not have to repeat the process for 1-4 years.

LIVER ISSUES
Sore / Tight / Stiff or Routine

Right Side of Neck?
Right Shoulder?
Right Arm?
Right Elbow or Upper Arm?
Right Upper Back
Headaches?
Insomnia?
Restless?
Poor Concentration or Memory?
Irritated Eyes?
Lung Issues?
Sinus Problems?
Skin Irritation?
Herpes?
Poor Digestion?
Exhaustion?
Hot Flashes?

For the full outline of organ symptoms reflecting their toxicity: read "Diagnostic Face Reading and Holistic Healing," 5th edition or later.

KIDNEY ISSUES
Sore / Tight / Stiff or Routine

Left Side of Neck?

Left Shoulder?

Left Arm?

Left or Right Wrist?

Left or Right Fingers or Thumb?

Mid Back?

Lower Back?

Hips?

Right or Left Buttock?

Right or Left Thighs?

Right or Left Knees?

Right or Left Calf?

Right or Left Ankle?

Right or Left Foot?

Cramps?

Heart Rhythm Issues?

High Blood Pressure?

Diabetes?

Frequent Urination?

For the full outline of organ symptoms reflecting their toxicity: read "Diagnostic Face Reading and Holistic Healing," 5th edition or later.

We are at war against purveyors of chemical addiction. They want us addicted to control our income. If they win, we are enchained servants for the rest of our lives.

Big Junk Food, Modern Medicine and its arm Big Pharma need us to be on five medications and to have had one surgery by age 30. Drugged minds do not consider using Natural Healing. A toxic body cannot execute routine maintenance, dooming it to fall short of its expected lifespan.

The confused are led by the loudest voice which is owned by Big Pharma, Modern Medicine and Big Junk Food. Addicting and injurious coffees and decaffeinated brews still hold 8 to 25% of their caffeine, we cannot win using them. The addicted; line up like sheep for another cup of caffeine or another energy drink. Caffeine is like a liquid computer virus attacking our immune system.

A desperate and dubious study was offered in 2012 laughingly claiming caffeine was good for everything from longevity to Alzheimer's. Do not believe such tripe. When sales of a product start to slip, it is not unusual for the financially strapped business, to purchase a study championing the wayward product's imagined value. Do not be duped.

Beware as you cannot win a game you do not know you are playing

Candy		Allergies
Breads or Flour of Any Kind	**Symptoms on**	Acne
Processed Gluten or Wheat	**the left often**	Breathing Issues
Pasta		Cravings for Sweets
Rice	**start out as**	Cravings for Junk Food
Crackers	**indulgences**	Poor Circulation
Cookies		Colds or Sick
Soy Products	**and bad habits**	Stress "Getting to you"
Cereals / Oatmeal / Pancakes		Temper or Poor Moods
Sweeteners	**on the right.**	Depression or Anxiety
Milk/ Cheese / Yogurt		Fibromyalgia
Processed Meat		All types of Arthritis
Caffeine an Any Type	**Eliminating**	Crohn's Disease or Bowel Upsets
White / Brown or Processed Sugar	**these is life**	Lupus or Immune System Upsets
Salt / Sodium		Liver issues including hepatitis
Decaffeinated Drinks & Green Tea	**and health**	Diabetes or Kidney Problems
Alcohol		Epstein Barr or Chronic Fatigue
Tobacco Products	**changing.**	Constipation or Leaky Gut
Medications or Drugs		Generally Exhausted or Worn-out
Junk / Frozen or Fast Food		Poor Sleep

Chapter 24 • Homemade Medicine

Disease and illness can best be described as toxicity on the rampage. The reasons we become ill are the factors of emotional stress releasing hormones overwhelming the body, intake of toxicity from meals, intentional chemical poisoning and accidental chemical poisoning.

No one is born broken, they may have limitations yet limitations are only problems for those who do not know what they are. All deciding to succeed against the odds can, if they put their mind to it. We therefore are only as limited or broken as we think we are, and no more than that.

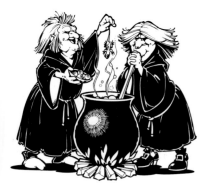

Before there was Modern Medicine there was Nature and its gifts. Those gifts are still with us if we know how to use them.

In the past medicines were brewed at home. Yes, herbs are excellent when eaten straight from the garden and they do heal. But, to make them a strikingly powerful immune system activating chemical, one that can awaken it from a toxic slumber, cooking is an amazing tool.

Medicines, herbals, Homeopathy & other methods of administering chemicals do not heal. Only an active immune system does that.

If medications or herbs healed, we would live indefinitely. The immune heals body, when it is shot, nothing can save us or we would live forever. We do not keep our immune system in a bottle on our nightstand.

Medicines have their place to alarm our immune system into action. Like an old wise healer we can learn to make medicine at home. The longer a mix is brewed the more powerful it becomes. Mom's chicken soup really was medicinal.

Coco Beans refined become chocolate. 7500 lbs. of Coca Leaves render 2 ½ pounds of cocaine. With this in mind, normal cooking renders mild drugs. This is where the phrase "The cure is in the kitchen" came from. This is also why so many are opting to become Raw Foodists as cooked food can make one ill.

Before we had medicine the wise woman or wise man often cooked up concoctions based on the above principals. The Witches of Shakespeare's Macbeth conjured medicines they called potions.

With a little experience and understanding of the process and practice, you can make homemade medicine. The details of how cooking creates drugs are detailed in "pH MADNESS."

Here are two simple homemade recipe' variants that produce huge results. You can season to your liking, but beware of too much salt.

Home Medicine Base

1 onion thin sliced	2 oz. of broccoli chopped
4 garlic sections chopped	2 oz. of cauliflower chopped
Juice of 1 lemon	2 oz. of green or red bell pepper

Mix one of the spice mixes below with the base above.

SPICE MIX #1

¼ teaspoon rosemary,	1/8 teaspoon of sea salt
¼ oregano	1/4 teaspoon parsley,
¼ dill weed	1/8 teaspoon of cayenne pepper

SPICE MIX #2

¼ teaspoon cilantro	1/8 teaspoon of cayenne pepper
¼ basil	1/8 teaspoon of sea salt
Pinch of cumin	¼ teaspoon of thyme

Sautee until garlic & onion are transparent. Add contents to 1 gallon of water & simmer for 2 hours. Eat a ½ cup every 1 to 2 hours until you feel better. *{All wanting a MEDICINAL chicken soup mix add 2 well-cooked shredded chicken thighs with their juices, simmer & serve.}*

Chapter 25 • **The Inner Body**

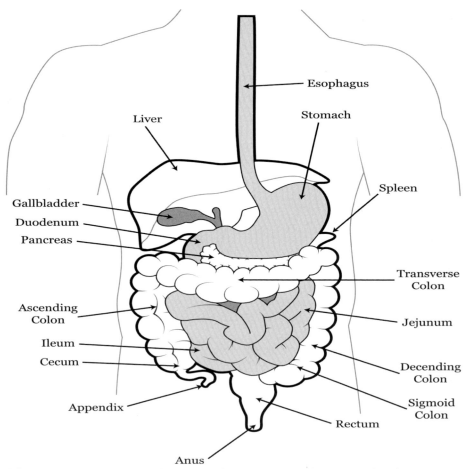

The most common toxins are white sugar, all types of salt, processed sodium, caffeine, tobacco and alcohol. These are not the only toxins, just the most common. In a polluted body the immune system is in a suppressed coma-like sleep. It snoozes as we absorb more & more toxins.

Detoxification awakens the immune system, enabling it to fight back.

Chapter 26 • Raw Food Meal List

9 AM Breakfast List

Breakfast offers the most time to digest before the end of the day. Because we have more time to digest, our heaviest foods can be eaten here. Most of the breakfast items listed here; need more digestive time. If you like, you can pull your breakfast meal from the lighter lunch list.

All lettuce	Snap Peas	Zucchini
Spring Mix	Jicama	Kale
Arugula	Tomato	Cabbage
Green Onion	Cucumber	Leeks
Onion White	Mint	Tomatillo
Garlic	Squash	Sweet Potato
Cauliflower	Corn	Radishes
Broccoli	Cilantro	Cilantro
Avocado	Beets	Celery
Radish	Basil	Asparagus
Bell Pepper	Carrots	Potato

Lunch List -12 NOON- Easy to Digest

Blueberries	Pineapple	Pears
Grapes	Apples	Cranberries
Oranges	Peaches	Star Fruit
Tangerines	Water Melon	Dragon Fruit
Grapefruit	Cantaloupe	Apricots
Pomelos	All Melons	Lemons
Kiwi	Papaya	Limes
Pomegranate	Plums	Loquats
Raspberries	Strawberries	Litchi nuts
Blackberries	Cherries	Jujube
Kumquat	Coconut wtr	Nectarines
Tomatoes	Mangos	Ugli Fruit

Snack List

The Snack list is chosen as all the items quickly digest and many of them are very beneficial for our main filters the liver and kidneys.

Blueberries	Raspberries	Cantaloupe	Cranberries
Grapes	Blackberries	Papaya	Star Fruit
Oranges	Kumquat	Plums	Dragon Fruit
Tangerines	Tomatoes	Strawberries	Apricots
Grapefruit	Pineapple	Cherries	Lemons
Pomelos	Apples	Coconut wtr	Limes
Kiwi	Peaches	Mangos	Nectarines
Pomegranate	Water Melon	Pears	Ugli Fruit

Dense Raw Protein List

Avocado: *1 med. 4.06 grams*
Sweet Potato: *1 med. 4.39 grams*
Potato: *1 med. 4.33 grams*
Corn Ear: *1 Large 4.02 grams*
Guava: *1 cup 4.21 grams*
Pomegranate: *1 med. 4.71 grams*
Blackberries: *1 cup 2.00 grams*
Broccoli: *1 cup 3.72 grams*
Cherries: *1 cup 1.46 grams*

Zucchini: *1 large 1.87 grams*
Cucumber: *1 large 1.75 grams*
Wheat Kernels: *¼ cup 6.5 grams*
Blueberries: *1 cup 1.1 grams*
Alpha Sprouts: *1 cup 1.32 grams*
Banana: *1 medium 1.29 grams*
Almonds: *¼ cup 8 grams*
Cauliflower: *1 cup 2.28 grams*
Tomato: *1 large 1.80 grams*

Raw Nut note: Raw nuts are not raw. They are blanched prior to being sold as raw. Blanching is cooking. Unless your raw nuts are purchased directly from a grower that you trust, avoid them.

Beware of HPP Juice. This stands for High Pressure Pasteurization, it is supposed to be RAW but it is not. HPP is pasteurized via 87,000 pounds of pressure per square inch. This creates intense heat quickly killing all life in the juice. The makers claim their juice is "Never Heated." That is true as they did not heat the juice; the pressure did the job DESTROYING it.

Digestive Challenging Foods

These food are best eaten in the morning

Broccoli	All Lettuce	Cucumber	Mustard Grns.
Cauliflower	Cabbage	Zucchini	Rutabaga
All Raw Nuts	Celery	Snap Peas	Chard
Bananas	Sprouts	Spinach	Leeks
Bell Peppers	Corn	Turnips	Thyme
Green Onions	Beets	Basil	Tarragon
Onions Carrots	Squash	Cilantro	Fennel
Radishes	Kale	Parsley	Sage
Asparagus	Ginger Rt.	Oregano	Mint

Liver / Kidney List

Liver Foods Include:
Blueberries, Raspberries, Romaine Lettuce, Tangerines, Oranges, Grapefruit, Lemons, Limes, Tangelos, Kumquats, Onions, Bell Pepper, Garlic, Apples

Liver Herbs Include:
Dandelion, Gentian, Yellow Dock, Irish Moss, Astragalus, Bupleurm, Hyssop, Saraparilla, Ginger, Thyme, Marshmallow, Garlic, Red Clover, Peony Root

Kidney Foods Include:
Grapes Tomatoes, Kiwi, Romaine Lettuce, Bell Pepper, Garlic, Cherries, Dragon Fruit, Beets, Raspberries, Coconut, Watermelon, Tomatillo, Loquat

Kidney Herbs Include:
Cinnamon Bark, Cedar Leaves, Wild Rose Root, Red Raspberry, Cayenne, Damiana Leaf, Holy Basil, Cloves, Goldenseal, Lycci Fruit, Juniper Berries, Fenugreek, Pygeum Bark, Borage Leaves

Chapter 27 • Raw Salad Dressings

These recipes are best made in a Vita Mix or good blender

Orange Basil Dressing
1/4 cup fresh squeezed OJ
4 basil leaves
1/4 of a bell pepper
Mix to a rough consistency

Suzy-Sierra Pepper Dressing
2 Large Bell Peppers
1 Orange
1/2 Pear
1 tsp. fresh chopped garlic
½ teaspoon of tarragon
1/8 teaspoon of black pepper
Blend to a semi-smooth consistency.

Oceanside Carrot Dressing
3 medium carrots
2 tsp. fresh chopped ginger
2 mint leaves
½ teaspoon of honey
1/8 tsp. coarse bl. pepper
Blend to a semi-smooth consistency.

High Protein Avocado Dressing
High Protein Avocado Dressing
1 large pitted avocado
1 Roma tomato
15 fresh basil leaves
1/8 cup of honey
1/8 cup reverse osmosis or spring water
Mix unt l smooth

Curry Coconut Dressing
¼ cup fresh (not canned) Coconut Water
¼ cup fresh coconut meat
2 basil leaves
1 mint leaf
2 teaspoon of fresh squeezed OJ
½ teaspoon Thai or Indian curry powder
¼ teaspoon cumin
¼ teaspoon of lime juice
Mix until smooth

Stacy Mango Dressing
2 medium tomatoes
1 large mango
¼ teaspoon tarragon
Mix until smooth

Appaloosa Papaya Dressing
1 papaya
1 steak tomato large
¼ green bell pepper
4 basil leaves
1 garlic wedge
1/8 lemon (section)
Blend until smooth

Stacy's Western Dressing
4 Roma tomatoes
1 freshly peeled lime
¼ Mango
20 Cilantro leaves
6 Oregano leaves or ¼ tsp. dry leaves
¼ teaspoon cumin
¼ Oregano
Blend until semi-smooth

Index

H
HCG, 62
Hunter Gatherers, 5
L
Lupus, 15, 38, 52, 96
M
Milk, 27, 63, 64, 65, 66, 77
mineral, 95,
Modern Medicine, 3, 4, 11, 35, 38, 52, 86, 87, 96
P
Paleo Diet, 54
protein, 17, 22, 42, 48, 49, 56, 57, 58, 59, 60, 81
R
Raw Food, 24, 33, 42, 43, 44, 45, 46, 47, 48, 49, 50, 52, 53, 54, 55, 57, 62, 63, 65, 67, 90, 91, 92
S
SNACKS, 49
T
toxins, 6, 44, 57, 67, 77, 78, 79, 81, 83, 89
V
vegetables, 5, 15, 79
veggies, 95
W
water, 6, 25, 26, 33, 37, 38, 40, 42, 46, 55, 56, 67, 68, 69, 70, 71, 75, 76, 77, 88, 95
World Health Organization, 31, 81

DISCLAIMER
This book asks you to determine based on your own testing and with the help of your Nutritionist and or medical professional, how to best improve your health. The Ancient Raw Food Diet is based on logic and testing. But only you can determine what is true or right for you. Be your own judge and jury and trust what you know to be true. You can be your best friend, if you trust yourself.

The repair cycles of the body are on a schedule that does not change. **PAGE 3**

Modern Medicine grips the planet in a strangle hold, via their maniacal drugs and greed. With use of brilliant double talk and chocking propaganda trumpeted by their media outlets, its blinding sales determination has paid off. They have amassed an empire almost incalculably vast. **PAGE 3**

What the last paragraph describes is a recipe' for heart attacks, strokes, leg cramps, brain fog, Lupus, Fibromyalgia, Chronic Fatigue, Crohn's, Wagner's, Hashimoto's, Epstein Barr, Mono, Osteoarthritis, Rheumatoid Arthritis, Arthritis, Post-Polio, Auto-Immune, Reynaud's, Shingles, Leaky Gut, Graves, Gilberts and even AIDs symptoms which can suddenly arise if the body is exposed to objectionable meals or wrong eating times. **PAGE 38**

Our worth at current estimation is 40 million US dollars for a life time of care. As this book is reprinted, add 1-2.5% a year for an approximation of our rising life time sickness value. **PAGE 38**

Waking at the same hour is vital as the body burns energy hourly and will weigh less an hour from now if you don't drink or eat anything. Waking at the same hour daily gives you an accurate measure of apples against apples. **PAGE 45**

No, all the fish on earth are not toxic with chemicals. If they were raised in a small pond under strict controls with no pesticides, they would be safe. Pond raised fish makeup less that 1% of all fish on the planet. **PAGE 75**

The idea of Free Radicals is science fiction. Free Radical; is a term that has been with us since the early 1900's. It simply means toxin. That is all a Free Radical is, it is just a toxin. Please substitute Toxin for Free Radical, thus putting it on the junk heap of confusing terms. **PAGE 83**